Pocket Psychiatry

Pocket Psychiatry

Kamaldeep Bhui, MSc, MRCPsych, DipClinPsych
Wellcome Training Fellow, Institute of Psychiatry,
De Crespigny Park, London and Honorary Senior Registrar,
Maudsley Hospital

Scott Weich, MSc, MRCPsych
Lecturer, Institute of Psychiatry, London

Keith Lloyd, MSc(Econ), MSc, MRCPsych
Senior Lecturer, University of Exeter, and
Consultant Psychiatrist, Exeter Community Trust

With contributions by Anne Aubin BM, MRCPsych
Senior Registrar in Child and
Adolescent Psychiatry, Plymouth

WB Saunders Company Ltd
London   Philadelphia   Toronto   Sydney   Tokyo

W. B. Saunders Company Ltd   24–28 Oval Road
London NW1 7DX

The Curtis Center
Independence Square West
Philadelphia, PA 19106-3399, USA

Harcourt Brace & Company
55 Horner Avenue
Toronto, Ontario M8Z 4X6, Canada

Harcourt Brace & Company, Australia
30–52 Smidmore Street
Marrickville, NSW 2204, Australia

Harcourt Brace & Company, Japan
Ichibancho Central Building, 22-1
Ichibancho, Chiyoda-ku, Tokyo 102, Japan

A catalogue record for this book is available from the British Library

ISBN 0-7020-2151-2

Typeset by Phoenix Photosetting, Chatham, Kent
Printed in Great Britain by
Mackays of Chatham PLC, Chatham, Kent

CONTENTS

Section V Liaison psychiatry

Section VI Working in the community

Section VII Special topics

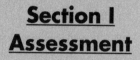

Section I
Assessment

THE PSYCHIATRIC ASSESSMENT

An overview of the necessary information from the history and mental state examination is presented below. This aims to serve as an *aide mémoire* for the commonest types of problem areas but is not comprehensive. A more detailed overview can be obtained from the major textbooks on psychiatry and psychopathology[1-3] and the descriptive psychopathology section (p. 347).

THE PSYCHIATRIC HISTORY

Basic information

Name, age, sex, first language, ethnicity, religion, address, telephone number, occupation.

Names and telephone numbers of:

- Any health care professional involved in care: GP, psychiatrists, psychologists.
- Any social services professionals involved in care: social worker, probation officer.
- Any voluntary organizations involved in care: housing, education, leisure.
- Family/friends who can provide immediate support and corroborative information.

Presenting problems

- According to patient.
- According to family.
- According to neighbours, friends, police, landlords, etc.

For each problem/symptom elicit:

Duration, onset, maximal/minimal intensity, periodicity, triggers

Aggravating factors and alleviating factors: classify as biological, social, psychological

Detailed account of most recent symptoms/problems which led to seeking help

Any evidence of depression, major psychoses, suicidality?

What interventions and coping strategies has the patient already used?

What interventions and coping strategies were unsuccessful and why?

Social circumstances

HOUSING
Cost, quality, crowding, contented?

EMPLOYMENT
Duration, stability, recent functioning

FINANCIAL
Income and debts

RELATIONSHIP
Married? Long-term partner? Any difficulties recently?

LIFE EVENTS
Bereavements, loss of work, stressors, relationship problems, any recent significant changes of circumstance

Family history

<u>4</u>

Family psychiatric diagnoses, contact with hospitals (medical and psychiatric), treatments used, current level of contact with index patient, current state of psychiatric illness, occupations, proximity. Identify any unexplained deaths, sudden death associated with alcohol, potential suicides and any evidence that relatives had a mental illness.

Relationship with siblings and parents, trusting relationships, any trusts broken? Closeness, amount of contact, effective social support provided? Separations – how were they managed?

Other children: ages, schooling, development, academic progress, illness – specific nervous problems, any evidence of conduct disorder, severe unhappiness – contact with social services, hospitals, GP.

Personal history

CHILDHOOD
Information from memory, family or reports. Early indicators of personality traits. Life events – unhappiness. Include physical illness, neurotic traits such as fears/phobia. Academic and social progress, special needs school? Truancy, school phobia, bullying, victimization for other reasons (obesity, race, size, etc.). Try to obtain old school reports, psychological assessments and any other source of data. Timing of school changes, reasons for, adjustments to changes, friendships

- Place and date of birth

- Family size and birth order

- Early childhood

- Childhood illness
- Developmental delays
- Schooling
- Changing school

ADOLESCENCE
Hobbies, ambitions, personality, life events, academic record, unhappiness, relationships, sexual experience, negotiating puberty and sexual development, relationship with peers, teachers, relatives and parents

ADULTHOOD
First job, length of occupations subsequently, reasons for change of job, problems with authority, colleagues, family and friends. Life events. Relationship successes and failures (include reasons for). List all major relationships, duration, specific problems, how they ended – any pattern? Marriages, children, sexual functioning during and between relationships, sexual victimization, sexual offences (if relevant) and fantasy life. Hobbies, sports, social, special skills, any achievements

- Employment
- Relationship
- Leisure

Past psychiatric and medical history

List past hospital admissions, operations, illness, treatments starting with most recent. Obtain records if possible from previous admission and treatment episodes. If information lacking contact previous Responsible Medical Officers (RMOs: the consultant-in-charge). Results from previous investigations can save much time and prevent unnecessary repeat investigations.

Personality

Elicit patient's self-report of strengths and weaknesses, how they start and end relationships. Ask about any good friends, did they have pets in childhood, did they have any meaningful relationships, how do they deal with frustration, anger, aggression, jealousy, episodes of sadness, low self-esteem? How does the patient perceive that others treat him/her? Criminality, special skills and abilities. Obtain informant history: GP, friend, partner, family member. Identify any maladaptive recurrent patterns of behaviour, when they arose and the negative consequences. Does the patient identify any aspects of their behaviour as problematic either for their social or occupational functioning? Is there any evidence that the patient can change their behaviour on the basis of previous experience? There are some simple structured instruments (often self-report) that will help with the assessment of personality (for example Ryle's 'Psychotherapy File').[4]

Medication

List all current medications, their indications, the side-effects that the patient experienced; previous medications and reasons for stopping. Record any drugs to which patient has had adverse or allergic responses. Note how reliably the patient can recall this information and how frequently and to what extent the patient varies their medication regimen.

Substances of abuse

Obtain detailed information about specific drugs used, the amount, the duration of effect, the adverse effects experienced, associated criminal activities, associated financial difficulties, the cost, escalation in use, contact with hospitals, administration routes, clean needle use. HIV/hepatitis B/C status. Previous treatment episodes in or out of hospital, detoxification strategies used. Specific names and addresses of doctors, therapists and clinics must be corroborated. Was the Home Office notified? Prescribed maintenance regimens? Every aspect of the history needs to be corroborated – drug craving and associated financial difficulties encourage addicts to obtain drugs by any means possible.

Forensic history

Identify any previous criminal convictions, the exact nature of the offence (e.g. weapons, injuries to self or others), any prison sentences served, duration of sentences, any psychiatric assessments at the time, ever diverted from court or prison to hospital under Mental Health Act order; were these regional secure units or district hospitals? Try to identify specifically courts, forensic psychiatrists and prisons where they were assessed.

MENTAL STATE EXAMINATION

APPEARANCE

Clothes (clean, old, inappropriate for weather, sexually revealing), smoking, gait, level of consciousness, coordination over limbs, mannerism, stereotypies, agitation, tremor and parkinsonian symptoms (bradykinesia, rigidity – cogwheeling), torticollis, dystonias, tardive dyskinesia, facial expression (frowning, sad, blunted, smiling, incongruent to emotions). Physical disabilities, scars, visible cuts on arms, needle marks visible, tattoos

BEHAVIOUR

Overactivity, underactivity, stuporosed, attacking others, able to hold conversation, frightened, staring into corners of the room, preoccupied by internal experience, perplexed, long pauses in answering questions, distractible, wringing hands, pacing around the room, sitting and then standing, invading personal space, sexually inappropriate, threatening, unpredictable

MOOD

Expansive, elated, grandiose, overfamiliar, laughing infectiously, irritable, angry, anxious; changes from depressed and responding to conversation to depressed and unable to engage in any conversation. Restricted range of emotional expression? Ability to feel remorse, presence of guilt. Do any preoccupations suggest depression (e.g. poverty, worthlessness, helplessness, morbid fears about body function)?

SPEECH AND THOUGHTS

Dysarthria or dysphasia – fluent or non-fluent (see ref. 3 for a detailed discussion of dysphasias). Comment on form, flow and content. Form: thought disordered, 'knight's move' thinking, flight of ideas, circumstantiality. Flow: pressure of speech, hesitant, interrupted by distraction, word-finding difficulties, logoclonia, echolalia. Content: neologisms, paraphasia, bizarre beliefs (see below), illogicality

Thought interference from outside agencies (thought insertion), thought blocking (snapping off; thought withdrawal), broadcast, fusion, muddling, concrete thinking, overinclusive thinking

PERCEPTIONS
Hallucinations (true and pseudo): visual, auditory, somatic, gustatory, olfactory. Hypnagogic, hypnopompic, functional, reflex, extracampine. Depersonalization, derealization, illusions, imagery

BELIEFS
Delusions: systematized, simple, monosymptomatic, or overvalued idea. Culturally sanctioned and religious beliefs can sometimes be misunderstood as indications of illness. If any unusual beliefs are elicited, evaluate how their reality may be tested. How does the patient respond to the suggestion that you wish to check out the details and evidence? How did these beliefs arise: what persuaded the patient that what they believe is true? How does the patient appraise evidence inconsistent with the content of the beliefs?

ANXIETY SYMPTOMS
Obsessional thinking, compulsive behaviour, panic attacks, phobic avoidance of places, people, animals, situations. Overaware of bodily functions. Observe sweating, tremor, fearful affect

PERSONAL EXPLANATION AND INSIGHT
Ask the following questions. Does the patient have any unusual experiences? Could these be

signs of illness? Has the patient's behaviour altered recently? Have any of their friends, family, church, etc. noticed this change? Has this change brought them into any conflict with people? Is the change desirable? Is it indicative of illness? Do any of the changes in thinking and behaviour constitute an illness which falls within the domains of psychological functioning? Do they need treatment for this illness? Will they accept treatment (physical, i.e. drugs; psychotherapeutic; social circumstances need to change). Finally, when prescribed treatments or interventions are arranged the clinician needs to make a judgement about how well the patient's actual adherence is reflected by their verbal reports about compliance

Cognitive assessment*

ORIENTATION: time, place, personal. Age, date of birth, floor, building, people around (who are they?)

ATTENTION AND CONCENTRATION: registration of information: ask patient to repeat a number; increase the number of digits until they can no longer do this. Most people can manage seven items. Repeat with a seven-item number or name and address

MEMORY: five minutes following registration, test memory of seven-item name and address (do not warn the patient that you are testing memory otherwise they will rehearse)

Remote memory: account of their life and major public events during their lifetime and news within the preceding weeks

Visual memory can be tested by asking patient to draw/copy certain shapes, hiding them and asking patient to reproduce them after 5 minutes

---

* For patients with neuropsychiatric disorders a much more thorough assessment is required (see ref. 5).

LANGUAGE: naming objects, fingers – nominal aphasia is an early sign of dementia

Give a written (needs to be read by subject) and verbal two and three stage command. This tests comprehension (receptive dysphasia?) but also whether sequences of activity can be carried out. Agraphia is an inability to write, alexia is inability to read.[6] From the subject's speech and conversation during the interview one can identify dysphasia and dysarthria

INTELLIGENCE: simple arithmetic or serial sevens; some idea of IQ can be obtained form historical reports (school or psychology)

SPATIAL AWARENESS: draw a clockface, place hands on it. Copying a star, cube, cat or abstract design. Can patient find their way around the ward, building, local area?

Testing CNS functions

FRONTAL LOBE TASKS: sequences of behaviour, e.g. place your fist on the table, now the edge of the hand and now the flat of the hand; repeat this and continue doing so (Luria's test). Ask for the same with the other hand. As in the mini-mental state:[7] take this piece of paper, fold it in half and place it on the floor. Ask for test to be done with both hands. Interpretation of proverbs also used. Verbal fluency also used: say as many words beginning with the letter T or name as many four-legged animals as possible. Apathy, lability of mood, poor motivation and loss of social graces, disinhibition, irritability, perseverative utilization behaviour, urinary incontinence are also indicative of frontal pathology. Inferior frontal gyrus lesion affects Broca's area causing non-fluent dysphasia

TEMPORAL LOBE TASKS: non-dominant lesion affects visual memory, e.g. prosopagnosia. Dominant lesion affects verbal memory and sensory deficits such as alexia, agraphia and aphasia arise. Receptive aphasia usually presents as word salad and indicates Wernicke's area lesion. Musical agnosia. Bilateral lesions cause amnestic syndromes

PARIETAL LOBE TASKS: aphasia, astereognosis, two-point discrimination (normally 2 mm at fingertips). Gerstmann's syndrome when a dominant lobe lesion: dyscalculia, left/right disorientation, finger agnosia. Loss of spatial awareness (drawing a star, etc.), dressing apraxia, hemi-neglect, altered body image (these usually with a non-dominant lobe lesion)

OCCIPITAL LOBE TASKS: cortical blindness, colour agnosia. Anton's syndrome (vertebrobasilar occlusion) causes loss of vision but a denial of the deficit

PHYSICAL STATUS

A brief selective physical examination should always be carried out if any of the history or mental state or patient's self-reported symptoms indicate the possibility of organic illness. The following summary is a quick overview of potential psychiatric presentation with underlying organic illness. The commonest physical disorders referred are delirium or CNS disease presenting with disturbed behaviour or depression.

Physical examination

HEAD AND NECK: blood stains, scalp lacerations, neck movements, evidence of head injury, facial symmetry, neck lumps, facial colour (pallor or flushing), jaundice, complexion, rash, lid lag, exophthalmos, squint, gaze palsies, visual fields. Cuts, bruises, oro-facial movement disorders

EYES: pupils: equal size, dilated (anxiety, anticholinergics) or pin-point (opiates). Examine fundi if any indication of poor sight, metabolic or arterial disorder or neuropsychiatric presentation

HANDS: nicotine stains, nail length and cleanliness, pitting (psoriasis), evidence of cardiovascular, respiratory or metabolic disorders (clubbing, small infarcts – one of the signs of subacute bacterial endocarditis, which may arise in injecting opiate addicts), koilonychia, rheumatoid nodules and osteoarthritis (Heberden's nodes; indicate possibility of chronic pain). Tremor

PULSE RATE: increased: anxiety, thyrotoxicosis. Low: hypothyroid states, β-blockers

RESPIRATORY RATE: anxiety, asthma, heart failure, traumatic chest injury

BLOOD PRESSURE: low due to anti-adrenergic effects of psychotropic drugs? Addison's disease. High and labile in neuroleptic malignant syndrome, Cushing's syndrome, pain, severe anxiety states

CHEST: cardiac heave, evidence of failure (raised jugular venous pressure, peripheral oedema), listen to lung bases, cardiac murmurs, third heart sound. Exclude pleural effusions or any thoracic cage damage. Exclude chest infection

LIMBS: tone, power, reflexes. Check arms and legs for injection sites, self-cutting scars, abscesses, wasting, bruising, injures, old fractures, major joint movements. Exclude cellulitis

HEIGHT AND WEIGHT

NOTE: gynaecomastia (neuroleptics, alcohol, other drugs?), body hair distribution (anorexia/pituitary deficit), spider naevi, porto-caval anastomoses (? alcohol use). Abdomen – palpate liver edge; constipation due to psychotropics not uncommon; urinary retention due to anticholinergic effects of psychotropics? Possibility of pregnancy? Possibility of urinary tract infection?

If there are any signs or symptoms suggestive of medical illness perform a thorough examination and obtain the necessary physical investigations. Do not prescribe a course of psychotropic drugs

INVESTIGATIONS

14

The following are commonly used investigations in psychiatry and should be considered if the clinical history is suggestive of organic illness. They should not be routinely ordered and are most likely to be of value in the elderly.

PSYCHOLOGICAL: behavioural analysis. Structured instruments to evaluate psychopathology, suicidality and aspects of personality and their response to interventions and over time

IQ ASSESSMENT: neuropsychological assessment if focal deficits identified or suspected

SOCIAL: further assessment of housing, finance, benefits, bus-pass availability, debts, family support, leisure and day care. Social services needs assessment

BLOOD: full blood count, urea and electrolytes, liver function tests, thyroid function tests, VDRL – in special circumstances HIV, hepatitis B, hepatitis C, blood alcohol, therapeutic drug monitoring (lithium, carabamazepine, phenytoin) and to check compliance in refractory cases (e.g. antidepressant levels), paracetamol and salicylate levels after overdose

URINE: drug screens, culture and sensitivity for infection, glucose dipsticks, pregnancy tests

X-RAY: after trauma or if systemic illness suspected on basis of history and examination: skull, chest, abdomen, limbs – after trauma

CT AND MRI: in neuropsychiatric presentations

EEG: in neuropsychiatric presentations

SUMMARIZING THE ASSESSMENT: FORMULATION

In view of the considerable amount of information elicited during a full psychiatric assessment, the ability to succinctly summarize this information in order to effectively communicate with colleagues is essential.

DESCRIPTION

- Brief statement about demographics and presentation with 'active problem' list
- Brief statement about relevant past psychiatric history and current treatment
- Brief statement about personal and family history of relevance
- Important mental state findings

DIAGNOSIS

Give the differential diagnoses along with findings in support or contradicting each of these diagnoses

EXPLANATIONS

Why this patient, why now and why in this manner? Indicate protective and vulnerability factors. Use a grid:

	Biological	*Social*	*Psychological*
Precipitating			
Predisposing			
Perpetuating			

ACCURACY AND LIMITATIONS OF ASSESSMENT

- Personality: yours and the patient's
- Communication/rapport
- Other sources of information
- Inconsistencies in account
- Cultural factors: linguistic difficulties, female psychiatrist preferred
- Family assessment

MANAGEMENT

- Present a *plan* for each of the problems identified
- Present a *timescale* for implementation and review of each intervention

- Present sources of *further information*
- *Precautions*: risk analysis and procedures to prevent suicide and other adverse outcomes
- *Engage* other agencies: voluntary/statutory, health/social
- List: name of keyworker and individuals involved, their contact addresses and telephone numbers
- List Mental Health Act status: appeals, dates of tribunals, manager's hearings

REFERENCES

1 Gelder, M.G., Gath, D. & Mayou, R. (1994) *Oxford Textbook of Psychiatry*. Oxford: Oxford Medical Publications.

2 Kendall, R.E. & Zeally, A.K. (1995) *Companion to Psychiatric Studies*. Edinburgh: Churchill Livingstone.

3 Sims, A. (1988) *Symptoms in the Mind. An Introduction to Descriptive Psychopathology*. London: Baillière Tindall.

4 Ryle, A. (1990) *Cognitive Analytic Therapy: Active Participation in Change*. Chichester: John Wiley & Sons.

5 Kopelman, M. (1994) Structured psychiatric interview: assessment of the cognitive state. *British Journal of Hospital Medicine* **52**, 277–281.

6 Lishman, W.A. (1987) *Organic Psychiatry*, 2nd edn. Oxford: Blackwell Scientific.

7 Folstein, M.F., Folstein, S.E. & McHugh, P.R. (1975) 'Mini-mental state'. A practical method for grading the cognitive state of patients for the clinician. *Journal of Psychiatric Research* **12**, 189–198.

Section II
Psychiatric
Emergencies:

a Problem-based Approach

THE ANXIOUS PATIENT

Anxiety is a symptom of many psychiatric disorders, but may also be a normal adaptive response to a hostile or threatening environment.

Symptoms

IDEATIONAL
Apprehension
Fear

SOMATIC
Dry mouth, difficulty swallowing
Palpitations
Flushing
Pallor
Hyperventilation
Tremor
Increased gastrointestinal motility
Chest pain
Backache, headache, fatigue
Diarrhoea
Urinary frequency
Paraesthesia

CHRONOLOGICAL
Episodic
Continuous
Stress related

BEHAVIOURAL
Avoidance
Rituals, e.g. checking
Startle response heightened
Hypervigilance
Poor concentration
Insomnia
Reduced libido

Clinical features

Psychological symptoms

Irritability, difficulty in concentrating (patient complains of poor memory), fearful anticipation, sensitivity to noise, a feeling of restlessness, repetitive worrying thoughts (ruminations). Appearance: strained, furrowed forehead, tense, tremulous, pale and sweating and tearful.

Physical symptoms and signs

Autonomic symptoms (see somatic symptoms above), sleep disturbance, muscular tension, overbreathing, tingling in fingers and peri-oral paraesthesia due to hyperventilation.

Differential diagnosis

Psychiatric

- Schizophrenia
- Mania
- Depression
- Generalized anxiety disorder
- Phobic disorder
- Panic disorder
- Obsessive–compulsive disorder
- Post-traumatic stress disorder
- Acute reaction to stress
- Adjustment reaction

Physical/organic states presenting as an anxiety state

- *Alcohol and drug withdrawal/intoxication*: restlessness, overactivity, disorientation, inability to register information, preoccupation with internal experience, fearful affect, lability of mood, sweating, tremor, visual hallucinations in delirium tremens, fits, diarrhoea, abdominal cramps, sensitivity to noise, hyperalgesia. Look for evidence of drug use (injection sites, abscesses, liver flap, tender liver with hepatomegaly). Raised γ-glutamyl transferase or mean corpuscular volume indicates chronic excessive alcohol use. Liver function tests may be deranged in alcohol misuse.
- *Dementia*: disorientation, registers information but 5-minute recall impaired (disorder of learning), nominal aphasia, constructional apraxia, often unconcerned with impairments unless cognitive testing culminates in a catastrophic reaction, absence of systemic disease, focal neurological signs may be present in multi-infarct dementia and dementia of Alzheimer type. Subcortical dementia distinguished by lack of motivation, affective changes, abnormal gait and posture, dysarthria, ataxia, tremor with a gradual onset in the absence of language, learning and calculating disabilities.
- *Thyrotoxicosis*: sweating, heat intolerance, check for goitre, tachycardia, tremor, lid lag and exophthalmos.
- *Hypoglycaemia*: hunger, sweating, tremor, fatigue, dizziness, fear and apprehension. Check for a history of diabetes; glucose dipsticks will quickly establish whether intravenous glucose is necessary.

- *Unstable angina.*
- *Phaeochromocytoma*: episodic sweating, headache, tremor and hypertension. Rare but life-threatening; episodic anxiety with hypertension; check fundi (normal if episodic hypertension), tachycardia, urine screening test for 4-hydroxy,3-methoxy mandelic acid (VMA) (detects about 85% of cases).
- *Carcinoid syndrome*: episodic hypertension, sweating and flushing. Urinary 5-hydroxy-indoleacetic acid (5-HIAA) elevated.
- *HIV*: men more than women, risk factors include intravenous drug use, gay and bisexual men and partners.
- *Multiple sclerosis*: lability of mood.
- *Intracranial tumours*: personality changes accompany these, lability of mood, aggression.

IMMEDIATE MANAGEMENT

- The acutely anxious patient will be very distressed. He/she and his/her family may insist that *you* do something.

- Ensure that hyperventilation is not due to a chest infection or traumatic chest injury; check the pulse and blood pressure. Hyperventilation can be helped by breathing in and out of a paper bag so as to raise the plasma $P\text{CO}_2$. It is a low plasma $P\text{CO}_2$ that is responsible for light-headedness, dizziness and paraesthesia.

- Calm the patient by removal from a busy casualty department to a quieter room. Reassurance and calm explanation that the symptoms are due to the physiological effects of adrenaline may be sufficient.

- Acutely anxious patients may be too distressed to listen and become irritable and terrified.

- Oral diazepam (5–10 mg) should be sufficient. If a severe anxiety state with marked motor overactivity, fear or a severe panic attack with loss of control then a slow (1 mg min^{-1}) intravenous injection of Diazemuls (5–10 mg) (higher risk of thrombophlebitis with i.v. diazepam) should abate the attack.

- Follow this with a discussion of the undesirable effects of benzodiazepines and an explanation and exploration of factors exacerbating the anxiety state. A behavioural treatment programme individually or in groups should be arranged as soon as possible. If this was a single attack it may not happen again.

- If panic disorder is diagnosed or anxiety is related to agoraphobia or obsessive–compulsive disorder, then the 5-HT reuptake inhibitors have been shown to be of value even in the absence of depressive symptoms. This can take several weeks to become effective (see pp. 303–304).

- Avoid the prescription of benzodiazepines and inform the GP of any action taken. This group is vulnerable to developing dependence.

THE HOSTILE PATIENT

The patient in this situation may be actively violent, threatening violence or have been violent. Violence may be directed at property or personnel. The aim is to gain control of the situation quickly, assess the aetiological factors involved and treat the patient if necessary.

Predictors of violent behaviour

RECENT VIOLENT BEHAVIOUR

PREVIOUS VIOLENCE: early account in childhood with fights at school, cruelty to pets, exposure to violence in formative years, severe emotional deprivation, imprisonment for violent offences (rape, murder, manslaughter)

CARRYING WEAPONS: knives or guns or use in previous incidents

SEX: men are consistently more violent than women

SOCIOECONOMIC STATUS: commoner in lower socioeconomic class and if fewer social supports

DISINHIBITING FACTORS: drug and alcohol intoxication, organic: head injury frontal lobe damage; violence less common with temporal lobe damage

IMPAIRED ABILITY TO REASON AND DEAL WITH FRUSTRATION: learning difficulties or psychiatric disorder, command hallucinations, paranoid delusions

AGGRESSION IN RESPONSE TO PSYCHIATRIC SYMPTOMS: psychomotor agitation, excitative stage after catatonia, manic excitement

DISSOCIAL PERSONALITY DISORDER

Differential diagnosis

Psychiatric disorders associated with violence

- Schizophrenia (especially paranoid schizophrenia)
- Mania (manic excited states)
- Depression (agitated)
- Personality disorder: antisocial, borderline, intermittent explosive
- Post-traumatic stress disorder
- Acute reaction to stress

Physical/organic causes

- *Delirium*: violence may occur during a delirious state if the patient is experiencing persecutory or threatening delusions or hallucinations. Look for fluctuating pattern along with altering level of consciousness. Repetitive violence associated with delirium may occur more often at night. Consider head injury; post-ictal confusional states may also present like this although violence and goal-directed activity is unusual in post-ictal states. Exclude physical causes of delirium in the elderly (see pp. 51, 192 and 198).

- *Drug and alcohol intoxication or withdrawal*: alcohol acts as a disinhibiting agent but alcohol withdrawal may result in delirium tremens. Milder states of withdrawal are characterized by increased sensitivity to noise and irritability. Chronic alcohol use may result in alcoholic dementia or acute encephalopathy due to hepatic failure or thiamine deficiency (Wernicke's encephalopathy). Alcoholic hallucinosis and delusional disorder related to alcohol use should be considered. Again paranoid beliefs and command hallucinations are associated with violence. Withdrawal states related to sedative dependence (benzodiazepines, barbiturates, heroin) result in overactivity and irritability with a lower tolerance to frustration. Acute psychoses may occur with amphetamine, cocaine or LSD use. Violence may occur in a disorganized way as a consequence.

- *Dementia*: hallucinations and paranoid beliefs can arise in the demented. Impaired reasoning capacity plus lower threshold for frustration.

- *Organic personality disorder*: emotional lability, irritability, outbursts of anger or aggression. Cognitive changes with suspicion. This may involve frontal lobe damage. Abnormal EEG may be present with temporal slowing.

IMMEDIATE MANAGEMENT

- Take as many details as you can when the patient is referred paying particular attention to predictors of violence. Use all sources of information (past notes, etc.) to make a quick assessment of dangerousness. Assess involvement of weapons and potential for violence, most severe offence and how recent.

- Clear the public and other staff from the area. If patient is armed do not tackle yourself, contact the police and ask them to disarm. Involve hospital security.

- Secure adequate numbers of experienced staff trained in control and restraint techniques. There should be one person per limb and one for the head. One other member of staff (usually the doctor) to administer medication. Establish clearly who is in charge of the situation.

- Try talking the patient down in a confident but non-confrontational manner. If unsuccessful or if more violence is threatened or ensues proceed to control and restraint techniques.

- Use an intramuscular neuroleptic (haloperidol 5–10 mg or droperidol 5 mg). If the patient has been exposed to neuroleptic medication previously higher doses may be required. Wait 20 minutes and if still necessary repeat the dose. Continue this process until rapid tranquillization is achieved. Use i.v diazepam as an adjunct (10–20 mg Diazemuls; diazepam is associated with a higher incidence of thrombophlebitis). If an intravenous line cannot be established use i.m. lorazepam 2–4 mg (do not use i.m. diazepam as it is erratically absorbed).

- Once 'made safe' exclude other causes of disturbance such as head injury, delirium (and causes thereof) or substance intoxication. *Note*: if alcoholic delirium tremens is the cause of the behaviour then neuroleptics may precipitate a fit as they reduce the fit threshold. Nurse individually with frequent measurements of pulse, blood pressure, temperature and neurology.

- Consider legal status. A Mental Health Act section for assessment may be indicated. If a clear diagnosis has previously been established and the patient has relapsed then a section 3 is appropriate. If a patient is violent a section is not required before you act. You can proceed under common law as you are acting in the best interests of the patient and the public.

- If an open ward is unsafe (for patients, staff or the public if patient absconds) then a locked ward or forensic unit may be required. Discuss this during a debriefing session with all the staff involved.

THE DEPRESSED PATIENT

A patient may complain specifically of depression but only about 20% of primary care attenders actually exhibit their distress in this way. It is more likely that the clinician considers the patient to be depressed and then evaluates other possible explanations so as to guide treatment choices. Careful assessment is necessary in order to elicit the symptoms and signs of depression.

Symptoms and signs

PHYSICAL SYMPTOMS: lack of energy, sleeplessness, aches and pain

MOOD AND FEELING STATES: fed up, bored, angry or irritable, anxious, panicky feelings, tension

BEHAVIOUR: avoid going out, self-neglect, not hungry, not eating and losing weight, checking compulsively (e.g. light switches are off, doors locked etc.), inactivity including sitting still for hours (may be stupor)

THOUGHTS – DELUSIONAL: of being punished, of wrongdoing, of committing terrible crimes, of rotting insides, of having no body

THOUGHTS – MORBID: of something dreadful about to happen, nothing to look forward to, of harm coming to self or family unless patient behaves in a certain way. Unable to stop worries

THOUGHTS – SUICIDAL: wants to die, has tried to hurt self, has tried to kill self, has plans to kill self. Worry about bodily functions. Feeling worthless and of no value to anyone

Poor memory, concentration and learning skills. Loss of interest in usual hobbies

Differential diagnosis

Psychiatric

- Major depressive episode
- Minor depressive episode
- Generalized anxiety disorder
- Obsessive–compulsive disorder
- Panic disorder
- Puerperal states: psychosis and depression
- Agoraphobia

Organic

- Alcohol or substance misuse
- Infectious disease: HIV, pneumonia, influenza, syphilis
- Endocrine disorder: Cushing's syndrome, thyroid disorder
- Neoplastic: pancreas, lung, cerebral
- Iatrogenic: prescribed medication
- Neuropsychiatric: dementia, epilepsy, stroke

IMMEDIATE MANAGEMENT

- The priority is to evaluate the degree of depression, the presence of suicidal thoughts and intent and the selection of the appropriate package of interventions. The interview should be carried out in a comfortable environment. Relatives often wish to be present while the patient is being assessed. This is usually fine but may prevent the patient from expressing their true feelings; preferably some time should be set aside to see the relatives separately. A selective physical examination will be of value if the history and specific symptoms are suggestive of an organic component.

- Depressed patients often take longer to think through and respond to questions put to them. Allow answers to emerge. Do not pressure the patient into responding. They will be unable to respond openly if a trusting relationship has not been established. Silences are often more uncomfortable for the clinician who may have other patients to see. A silence for the depressed patient will give them the time to convey much of how they are feeling.

- In the presence of suicidality the extent of it should be assessed in detail (see pp. 33 and 198). If the patient is depressed and suicidal or at risk of serious self-harm, admit them for assessment. Night sedation is necessary if there are overt symptoms of anxiety and agitation. If possible and usually in the absence of an immediate threat to life the option of a return home under the supervision of a friend or relative may be arranged as long as the depressive symptoms are *actively managed*. Involve the patient's GP and make an outpatient appointment for the patient to see the psychiatrist.

32

- Sending a patient home with antidepressants without a proper assessment of suicide risk, or arrangements to monitor depressive symptoms at least weekly in the early stages may lead to a completed suicide. If there are social indicators of higher suicide risk, avoid sedative antidepressants. Use one of the selective serotonin reuptake inhibitors (SSRIs), which are less dangerous in overdose.

- Interventions directed at social and psychological factors in the aetiology and maintenance of depression should be identified and offered to the patient, e.g. improved housing, refuge for victims of violence etc. Involve the duty social worker early. Specific depressive beliefs, including contemplating suicide, are amenable to cognitive therapy. This skill can be exercised in the emergency situation to (1) identify depressogenic beliefs which can later be targeted by cognitive therapy, (2) evaluate the fixity of the beliefs, (3) to shift the target beliefs (suicidal thoughts) as part of acute treatment and assessment.

THE SUICIDAL PATIENT

Suicidality refers to deliberate and potentially fatal acts of self-harm. Suicidal thoughts are part of depressive symptomatology but can arise in any of the psychiatric disorders and should be specifically enquired about during assessment. The exact thoughts, feelings and actions of the patient must be identified and recorded in as much detail as possible.

Symptoms and signs

MOVEMENTS – DEPRESSIVE: psychomotor retardation, stupor, absence of reactivity of expression. Agitation, irritability, impulsive behaviour with or without violence to property or other people

MOVEMENTS – MANIC: consider manic excitement as part of a mixed affective state

THOUGHTS – DEPRESSIVE: slowing, or absence of any thinking. Worthlessness, hopelessness, helplessness, wish to escape from torment, wish to join dead relatives, wish to die as the most suitable punishment, wish to die as the only solution to social and relationship problems, wish to die for no obvious identifiable reason. May be accompanied by wish for punishment and guilt, of wrongdoing, of complete poverty (financial or physical, e.g. 'I have no heart' as part of nihilistic delusions)

THOUGHTS – PSYCHOTIC: delusions of immortality/being God and therefore able to be re-born, of taking one's life before persecutors (the devil, MI5, neighbours, etc.) do so

SEVERITY INDICATORS:
Evidence of careful planning
Previous attempts

Psychiatric diagnosis – recent visit to GP or psychiatrist

Chronic physical illness (pain; terminal illness)

Serious attempt

Violent method chosen

Family history of psychiatric disorder

Social/life events – bereavement, unemployment

Male

Elderly (rising incidence in young men and young Asian women)

Single

No support networks

Clinical features

Deliberate self-harm: repeated acts of non-fatal self-harm with no intention to die must be distinguished and can arise as part of acute distress states (bereavement, separation from partner, end of a relationship, social stressors) or from persistent conditions such as anxiety states, eating disorders, personality disorders and depressive states in schizophrenia or manic depressive illness. Affective symptoms can occur in isolation or as part of these syndromes.

Differential diagnosis and associated disorders

Psychiatric

- Affective disorder (including bipolar)
- Schizophrenia
- Persistent anxiety states
- Personality disorder: dual diagnoses

Organic

- Alcoholism: associated depression and social problems
- Substance misuse: social adversity, homelessness, financial problems, unbearable withdrawal symptoms
- Epilepsy: persistent
- Chronic disabling physical illness: loss of limbs, nervous system disorder
- Chronic pain
- Terminal illness: cancer

IMMEDIATE MANAGEMENT

- If the patient has taken an overdose or there is a open wound requiring immediate attention after self-injury ensure that this is attended to first. If another team (medical or surgical) take over the immediate care ensure that they are fully aware of the suicidal potential and that the patient is adequately emotionally supported and supervised before a detailed assessment can be carried out.

- If the patient is refusing life-saving treatment: explain carefully the risks of not having treatment, name the consequences and the timescale for them to take place, and explain the impact of treatment immediately or of delayed treatment. Evaluate their *capacity* to make an informed decision: they must understand the nature and consequences of their choice and *you* must be satisfied that they are able to appraise the information put before them. Record your assessment of capacity. If they do not have the capacity to make an informed choice treat under common law. Physical treatments cannot be sanctioned by placement on a detention order under the Mental Health Act. If the patient is trying to leave or is likely to injure themselves again or has harmed themselves they should be detained (pp. 96, 97 and 101).

- Until this is enacted it is essential that the patient be detained in their own best interests. In this situation clearly identify which nursing team (accident and emergency, ward) will be providing continuing supervision (24 hours).

- Involve and inform family members. They may be invaluable in helping persuade the patient to receive treatment. If the patient has not taken an overdose and has not harmed themselves, assess their immediate suicidal intent.

- Interview: establish rapport. Do not be afraid about asking questions about suicide

  Do they still want to die?

  What are their thoughts about the failed attempt?

  Are they likely to do this again?

  Do they have a detailed plan?

  Is the chosen method lethal?

  Did they allow for the possibility of being saved?

  Will they have the opportunity to enact the plan?

  Have the precipitating circumstances been resolved?

  Had they organized all their affairs in anticipation of a completed suicide?

  Was depression recently diagnosed?

  Were they prescribed some medication?

  What other interventions have been tried?

  Were any specific interventions helpful?

  Who would they go to for help?

  Would they see their GP?

  If discharged what measures are in place to prevent a recurrence?

  Would they consider drug treatment?

  Would they consider psychotherapy?

  If severely depressed would they consider electroconvulsive therapy (ECT)?

- If the *risks remain high* and there are no community interventions available or acceptable to the patient consider admission. If there are clear signs of depression (see p. 210) or social factors which are not immediately remedied, consider admission either for the safe treatment of depression in a protected environment under supervision or to intervene in the crisis.

- Admission under a section of the Mental Health Act may be especially necessary if (1) the patient expresses inconsistent views about their wish to remain voluntarily or return home, (2) there is a high likelihood of absconding, (3) there is the possibility of a fatal suicide attempt.
- Communicate the observation requirements to the nursing staff. Once on the ward ensure the patient is adequately supervised and record the level of observations necessary after a consensus is agreed with the nursing staff. If the patient is depressed but does not need admission: this finding will be the conclusion of a careful assessment which determines that the patient is not acutely suicidal or that their suicidality has abated as a result of social and psychological interventions delivered there and then, e.g. arrangements for accommodation, help with financial problems, providing further support by telephone availability and an outpatient appointment or home visit.
- Beware: denial of suicidal intent, impulsive distress, anger, malignant alienation, assumptions of improvement in the absence of evidence, poorly planned and coordinated treatment regimens[1] and repeated self-harm[2].

THE PERSONALITY DISORDERED PATIENT: A CAUTIONARY NOTE

The diagnosis of personality disorder is a difficult one to make on one interview. The term is used widely by professionals and the public often inaccurately. This section aims to identify the types of presentation in which personality disorder is the predominant factor, yet it is most likely to occur as a secondary diagnosis to other psychiatric conditions. A corroborative history is required before making a definitive diagnosis.

Clinical presentations

Aggression to staff or public

Demanding prescriptions – for self or to market on the street

After street brawl

Intoxicated – withdrawal states

Homelessness and demands for housing yet not taking up offers of what is available

Threats of self-harm – actual self-harm as a public display

Accusations of abandonment by services, family, partners

Presenting in crisis yet not accepting help or not adhering to any structured plan

Partners or children are presented – Munchausen syndrome (see p. 54)

Presents with physical symptoms in order to enter the sick role

Brought by police

Criminality – opinion sought urgently

Making the right decision

40

You cannot ignore this population. The fact that some patients are unpleasant can influence your judgement in favour of dismissing them. These presentations can arise from a diverse number of distinct disorders ranging from depression to schizophrenia to pure dissocial personality disorder and criminality. People with a personality disorder have a higher risk than the general public of suicide and in view of their inability to maintain successful relationships or social circumstance are likely to develop psychiatric disorders. Patients in distress may act in a manner that recruits from onlookers the label of personality disorder. Distressed people may behave in maladaptive ways and their coping strategies become more extreme. A crisis ensues when their strategies are increasingly unsuccessful.

Careful assessment, with information from relatives and friends as well as past health and social service contacts, is essential. If these people or agencies cannot be contacted immediately make another time to meet with the patient explaining the need to obtain as much information as possible. This is especially important in instances where prescriptions for controlled drugs are being sought. Always discuss your assessment with a senior colleague and record your concerns and the reasoning behind your conclusions and management plan.

Where there is sufficient information to make a diagnosis of personality disorder or where the demands of the patient are escalating and unreasonable making such a diagnosis more likely, *consider the possibility of a psychiatric disorder, the risk of suicide and violence to others*. If after an assessment meeting there is no evidence of a psychiatric disorder then admission is contraindicated. It will only reinforce maladaptive illness behaviour. Make it clear that although admission is not deemed necessary you will secure help in any other way and arrange for the patient to be seen again. If there are any potential social interventions that can be arranged, do so. This may involve urgent liaison with social services or a referral. Psychotherapy should be considered and if the patient is agreeable an assessment session for suitability booked as soon as possible.

Where the patient is complaining of physical illness and yet there are obvious signs of personality disorder, do a physical examination or arrange for the medical team or A & E staff to review him/her depending on level of urgency. If the history or presentation does not make sense or is incomplete and there remains a risk of self-harm or of serious physical illness as yet undetected, an admission for assessment will be necessary. This should be arranged after *careful discussion with nursing staff and the RMO*. If there are any concerns about violence or substance misuse whilst on the ward an admission contract may prevent the matter arising in crisis. Think of all the possible problems that might arise and record a management plan for each.

Assessment checklist

Psychiatric disorder?

Physical illness?

Substance misuse?

Violence potential?

Acting out potential if admitted?

Psychotherapeutic interventions?

Any success experiences: work, hobbies?

Intelligence and ability to tolerate frustration?

Suicide risk?

Any meaningful relationships?

Previous interventions (especially failed ones)

Management plan: disseminate to colleagues

THE HALLUCINATING PATIENT

Hallucinations are perceptions in the absence of a stimulus and can arise in any modality. The commonest are auditory, visual and somatic hallucinations. True hallucinations appear to arise in external space and have the quality of a perception following a stimulus. The prevalence and significance of hallucinations appears to vary across cultures.

Symptoms and signs

AUDITORY

Distractibility, inaccessibility, incongruent affect

Sudden changes of mood – fear, elation, giggling

Sudden changes of posture as if listening

Requests for silence

Holding a conversation with voices – whispering to self

Inability to think clearly

Occasionally no evidence of voices – disclosure after assessment

In second or third person, command or commenting

VISUAL

Looking into corners of the room

Sudden changes in affect – pleasure to terror, fear and depression

Usually associated in organic conditions with clouding of consciousness

Pulling at clothes or objects
Inability to get attention (usually with delirium)
Of people, faces, animals, scenes (fires of hell and the devil)
Note: people with little sight can hallucinate visually

SOMATIC
Sensations can arise in any part of the body – mouth, head, genitals; attribution of sensations to passers-by can lead to assaults

Clinical features

Visual hallucinations: distinguish from eidetic imagery when patients can voluntarily set off scenes that are vivid. Otherwise imagery is less vivid and has quality of not being real. Dim lighting potentiates illusion formation: emergence of images out of shapes, colours, form of real objects. Visual hallucinations more commonly arise in organic states. Auditory hallucinations may also arise in organic states but in this instance the voices are fragmented and transitory; other signs of organic states help distinguish psychiatric states from organic ones. Distinguish from pseudohallucinations in which the perception is not as real and seems to arise from within the person. Pseudohallucinations are usually ego-syntonic whereas true hallucinations are usually ego-dystonic. Hallucinatory experiences can fall within the realm of culturally sanctioned phenomena and hence are not always a sign of illness. Discussion with the patient's cultural reference groups will highlight if the experience is culturally inconsistent with health.

Differential diagnosis

44   Psychiatric

- Schizophrenia
- Major affective disorder: depression or mania with psychosis
- Brief psychoses and dissociative disorders
- Puerperal psychoses

Organic

- Alcoholic hallucinosis and drug intoxication withdrawal
- Dementia
- Delirium and metabolic disorders
- Temporal lobe epilepsy
- Tumours (CNS)
- Eye or retinal disease

IMMEDIATE MANAGEMENT

- The management of the hallucinating patient should focus on the exclusion of an organic disorder (see pp. 51, 192 and 198). Those with unexplained visual hallucinations should have an assessment of their visual fields and an ophthalmological examination. Pre-existing eye disease may facilitate the emergence of visual phenomena. Similarly the hard of hearing may have auditory hallucinations and middle ear disease should be excluded especially if the presentation is atypical. The assessment aims to make a confident psychiatric diagnosis and management plan on the basis of a history and psychopathology.

- Patients may be frightened and agitated. Poorly lit, noisy areas may exacerbate their fear. Remove the patient to a calm environment. Engage them in conversation and examine to what extent their functioning is impaired by hallucinations. During the course of a conversation signs and symptoms might spontaneously arise. Detailed questions about hallucinations are unlikely to result in immediate answers and it may take time to enable the patient to feel comfortable. Allaying some of their fear may be a necessary prerequisite. There is often a conviction amongst staff that some patients are hearing voices but on direct questioning they will deny it. Identify which of the features above are present and support the view that the patient is hallucinating. Some patients with persistent symptoms and in continuing contact with psychiatric services do not wish anyone to know of their hallucinations for fear of enforced treatment. Others may not be able to disentangle specific hallucinations from their range of abnormal experience. This assessment is made especially complex in individuals who have a limited pre-morbid capacity for communication: those with learning difficulties, head injuries, children, stroke victims, partially sighted, hard of hearing, etc. The management of individual patients is that of the primary diagnosis. Neuroleptic medication is of value in both organic and non-organic hallucinations. Generalized anxiety-relieving measures as discussed on p. 22 are of value in the acute situation. If anxiety is very prominent a benzodiazepine (diazepam 5–10 mg p.o.) should be given in addition to a neuroleptic (haloperidol 5–10 mg p.o.); if sedation is required use 50–200 mg chlorpromazine depending on body mass of patient (monitor blood pressure). If the patient is acutely disturbed and effective communication cannot be established then enforced sedation will be necessary (see p. 27).

- If the presentation is atypical and there are difficulties with obtaining a complete assessment (different culture, deaf, learning difficulties) avoid neuroleptics and any other medication if possible until a full assessment as an inpatient is completed.

THE PARANOID PATIENT

The term 'paranoid' is loosely applied to those who feel persecuted but in a psychiatric sense refers also to presentations of which the content is self-referential. A variety of self-referential symptoms can arise in the context of many of the major psychiatric disorders as well as a range of organic states.

Symptoms and signs

PERSECUTORY DELUSIONS
Neighbours, strangers, family members either torment or are watching or are responsible for a series of adverse events. Organizations or large institutions (real or delusory) may be held responsible for their distress

PERSECUTORY HALLUCINATIONS
Influence the content of delusional beliefs: 'we'll kill you … we will get you … you did it'

GRANDIOSE DELUSIONS
Having a special skill, role or mission in the world especially when there are elaborate beliefs about why the patient was chosen

MORBID JEALOUSY
Conviction that partner is having affair – checks partner's clothes, movements. Denial is interpreted as proof but if through frustration a confession is made, this only leads to exacerbation of the mental state. Patients are potentially dangerous as they may resort to violence. Morbid jealousy is associated with alcoholism and is commoner in men. It can arise in organic states

EROTOMANIA
Typical account is of a woman who falls in love with an unattainable man of higher status. All

acts by the man are interpreted to be consistent with his love being returned to her. Actions by the object of adoration even if openly discouraging or bluntly negative are interpreted as signals of the person's true but discreet love for the patient

SHARED DELUSIONS

When two people present with an unusual story it is often adopted as reality but in cases of induced psychoses two or more people living in isolation from others can develop a shared delusional belief which is self-referential and/or persecutory. In 90% of instances those sharing the belief are family members (sisters are commonest, followed by husband and wife, mother and child, two brothers, brother and sister, father/child, and unrelated)

SENSITIVE PERSONALITY TRAITS

In personality disordered – sense of injustice and prejudice, sensitive to any potential criticism. It may be difficult to distinguish severe paranoid personality disorder from paranoid psychoses

Differential diagnosis

Psychiatric

- Schizophrenia
- Affective psychoses: persecutory and self-referential symptoms
- Paranoid personality disorder
- Borderline states
- Severe acute distress: brief reactive psychoses
- Induced psychoses: may be persecutory

- Morbid jealousy (Othello syndrome): more self-referential than persecutory
- Erotomania (de Clérambault's syndrome): self-referential

Organic

- Drug-induced states: alcohol, cocaine
- Dementia
- Delirium

IMMEDIATE MANAGEMENT

- The background history is essential as the patient often appears to be able to hold brief conversations without obvious evidence of abnormality. Only when the specifics of his/her beliefs are examined along with accounts from third parties does the true picture emerge. This is why shared delusions are especially difficult to identify.

- The cultural context of beliefs should also be understood or at least evaluated by recruiting someone from the same culture before labelling beliefs as delusional. Substance misuse and organic conditions must be excluded.

- Bizarre mood-incongruent beliefs and hallucinations are likely to suggest schizophrenia whereas mood-congruent symptoms are more suggestive of affective psychoses (see p. 209). Brief reactive psychoses arise suddenly and often have an admixture of affective as well as confusional symptoms (p. 51).

- If a diagnosis of affective psychosis or schizophrenia is made, neuroleptic medication will have a role to play in the acute management of distress and disturbance. If, however, the diagnosis includes one of the self-referential and more unusual disorders, the prognosis is poor and separation from the object of the patient's belief or (in the case of shared delusions) from the sharer is the only safe treatment. With Othello and de Clérambault's syndromes there is a risk of violence by the dissatisfied patient. Love turns into grief and may become irritability and anger. Advise the object of attention that immediate separation is necessary and possibly an injunction; advise of the dangers of not doing so and of there being no immediate treatment.

THE CONFUSED PATIENT

Confusions refers to objective signs and subjective symptoms suggestive of impaired ability to think clearly. It is not itself diagnostic but raises the possibility of specific organic and non-organic disorders.

Symptoms and clinical features of confusion

Diagnosis	Delirium	Dementia	Non-organic
History	Sudden onset	Insidious	Either
Duration	Short (days)	Long (months)	Either
Conscious level	Impaired	Normal	Either
Course	Fluctuates	Progressive	Either
Disorientation	++ → +++	+ → +++	Either
Impaired registration	+++	0 → +	0 → +
Affect	Terrified Anxious Irritable	Indifferent Labile	Elation/depressive Labile/terrified
Psychomotor	Poverty Overactivity	Normal	Either
Sleep	++ → +++	0 → ++	Either
Reversibility	Often	Rarely	Often
Poor memory Short-term memory impairment	Not testable	+++	0 → +
Long-term memory impairment	Not testable	+ → ++	0
Speech	Rambling/ incoherent	Aphasia	Formal thought disorder, flight of ideas, mute Depressive content Anxiety
Focal neurology	0 → ++	0 → +	0
Focal cognitive signs	0	+ → +++	0

Differential diagnosis

Psychiatric

- Schizophrenia
- Brief reactive psychoses
- Depression (pseudodementia)
- Severe anxiety
- Dissociative state (fugue/conversion symptoms)
- Ganser's syndrome
- Munchausen syndrome

Organic

- Delirium (see p. 198)
- Dementia (see p. 192)
- Space-occupying lesions
- Epilepsy (simple or complex partial seizures or post-ictal confusion)

IMMEDIATE MANAGEMENT

- This will largely depend on whether the cause of confusion is delirium, dementia or a non-organic disorder. Exclude an organic cause. Delirium can be a sign of a medical emergency. Delirious patients may be hallucinating and expressing unusual beliefs that can be mistaken for frank psychosis. The fragmentary and transient nature of the symptoms along with poor registration would support such a diagnosis. Information is often difficult to elicit and corroborate.

- Management should be directed by physical examination and history but will often include obtaining information from an informant about past physical and psychiatric disorders, existing medication and checking full blood count, urea and electrolytes, liver function tests, glucose, thyroid function tests, B_{12} and folate. Also consider a drug screen, chest X-ray, ECG, EEG and CT scan. Blood cultures and lumbar puncture are indicated if there is an unexplained temperature or fluctuating conscious level indicating a possible cerebral infection.

- If a dementia is suspected an informant history is invaluable but a good cognitive assessment looking for focal deficits will help formulate a correct diagnosis. Lewy body dementia may present with recurrent delirious episodes. Focal neurology or seizures are suggestive of Alzheimer's disease. Lability of mood and disinhibition may be present in Pick's disease or any frontal lobe pathology. Reversible causes of dementia should be excluded. Immediate management may be directed to assessing the causes of socially embarrassing or hostile behaviour or dealing with immediate accommodation. People who have a dementia are more likely to present with delirium because of concurrent physical illness.

- The non-organic disorders include apparent memory impairment due to poor concentration accompanied by psychosis, severe anxiety or acute distress.

- Brief reactive psychosis, especially amongst certain cultural groups, may involve an apparent change in conscious level. Such states are of short duration and may resolve with supportive counselling, psychotherapy and/or benzodiazepines (rather than neuroleptics). Dissociative states are especially difficult to assess in view of the conspicuous absence of any form of identification. A small proportion of people presenting with apparent loss of memory may be ultimately diagnosed as having hospital addiction (Munchausen syndrome) or a Ganser syndrome-like state (somatic conversion symptoms, approximate answers, clouding of consciousness and pseudohallucinations). The degree of conscious motivation is the subject of much debate and should be considered after a comprehensive assessment with as much corroborated information as possible.

- If the non-organic diagnosis remains uncertain do not medicate, and assess for symptoms of physical and psychiatric illness, ability to have needs met, ability to interact with other patients and staff and ability to concentrate. Ensure neurological and cardiorespiratory observations and drug screen and sleep chart are completed. If a dissociative mechanism is suspected then abreaction, once established on a ward, will be the treatment of choice.

- If there is a risk of deliberate self-harm or unpredictable behaviour ensure adequate supervision is available with emergency medications if necessary (see p. 27). Consider legal status: if unable to give informed consent and a mental illness is suspected then an assessment for a Mental Health Act section should be arranged. If physical illness is significant then assessment and treatment should be carried out under common law with a clear documented assessment of competency to give consent to treatment.

THE POLICE-ESCORTED PATIENT

The police, in accord with Health Circular 66/90, are encouraged to divert the mentally ill to hospital at an early stage. They may accompany an individual because there is a history of mental illness or of suspected mental illness or the individual has sustained significant physical injuries. A psychiatric assessment may be requested by the casualty officer. Domestic violence may be a factor.

Symptoms and clinical signs

VIOLENCE
Note: Section 136; has patient been charged; offence details; handcuffs necessary? struggling? how many police officers? physical injury sustained by patient and police? accompanying threats of assault or actual assault; nature of inflicted injury or property damage; method used (physical aggression with hands, weapon used, fire involved); ability to hold a conversation calmly; staring with fixed eye contact; invasion of personal space

PSYCHOSIS OR ODD UNEXPLAINED BEHAVIOUR
Hallucinations: distractible, unpredictable, sudden activity, inaccessible periods, second person command hallucinations, persecutory hallucinations. Delusions: grandiose and omnipotent; are actions based on delusional role? Persecuted with fearfulness and escape behaviours

INTOXICATION
Alcohol on breath, disinhibited, fits, blackouts, delirium tremens, dysarthric, needle marks, charge involves handling substances

SUICIDE ATTEMPT

Ask the following questions. Where was patient picked up? Caught about to jump off a bridge? Wandering into traffic, on railways lines or the underground? Having inflicted injury on themselves in a public place? Following report of self-injury? Aggression? Why were ambulance staff unable to bring patient? Drowsy but with obvious account of self-harm or evidence of self-injury. Cuts on arms, neck, abdomen, genitals, etc. Bottles of psychotropic and other drugs found when picked up

HOMELESS

Homelessness may compound other problems. It may be the reason for self-harm, fearfulness, or it may have followed a mental illness with a gradual decline in self-care skills; hygiene, clothes appropriate for weather, nutrition, chest infection or tuberculosis?

UNRESPONSIVE

Consider fugue and stupor. Found wandering; personal identifications absent, not responding to questions, mute or withdrawn. Amnesia

Differential diagnosis

Psychiatric

- Schizophrenia: first episode or relapse
- Paranoid psychosis
- Bipolar affective disorder: depressive episode (syn: major depression)
- Bipolar affective disorder: manic episode
- Personality disorder
- Dementia
- Fugue
- Learning difficulties

Organic

- Alcohol intoxication/withdrawal
- Other intoxication/withdrawal states: cannabis, cocaine, amphetamine, LSD, solvents
- Delirium
- Head injury
- Post-ictal

IMMEDIATE MANAGEMENT

- The police should contact the duty psychiatrist and the approved social worker (ASW) as soon as they place anyone on a section 136. Alert casualty staff, and the person responsible for identifying a bed should the patient need admission. On arrival check the legal status: section 136 or 135 or informal. The ASW should see the patient whether detained or not. If there are grounds for detention it is good practice to implement a section for admission (section 2 or 3) as soon as possible rather than admit a patient on a section 136. Two section 12 approved doctors need to be sought (or the patient's GP and one section 12 approved doctor; see pp. 96–100). As soon as you have satisfied yourself of the need for formal admission ensure the doctors and ASW are aware and identify when they will do a joint assessment. If the patient is to be admitted informally then the section 136 ends once the ASW has assessed the patient. Obtain as much information from the police about any offence and the circumstances of their involvement. If charges are to be dropped then ask the police to remain with the patient until your assessment of dangerousness is complete. You may have to ask for assistance from hospital security.

- Ensure that any obvious or severe injuries that require immediate attention are addressed by the casualty team. Ensure that the staff and assessment environment is safe. If in doubt ask for nursing staff or the police to remain with you during the assessment. Similarly before asking for handcuffs to be removed ensure that the assessment room is comfortable, alarmed, and will prevent absconding. Document the time each stage of the assessment is completed.

- Before the assessment of the patient quickly review past records and consider dangerousness, suicide risk, most recent mental state assessment, identified team providing care, previous treatments and reasons for relapse. Identify past criminal record, psychiatric history, substance misuse history, past incidents of violence and any physical illness.

- The assessment: learning difficulties and ability to communicate effectively, current suicide intent and most recent attempt, nature of offence, weapons used, intention to harm others, reasons for harming self or others (based on delusional beliefs or in response to hallucinations). Specific psychopathology which may help narrow the differential diagnosis. A cognitive assessment performed at this stage may be invaluable should subsequent court reports be required but also is essential to exclude dementia and may allude to the possibility of a fugue state. Document the patient's detailed account of events and especially their reasons for committing the offence paying attention to ability to recall details of the event, bizarre explanations, illogical answers, remorse, regret, frequency of carrying weapons, competency to give consent for any treatment offered. The reason given leading up to and after the offence warrants careful scrutiny and if unusual or suggestive of mental illness an assessment admission should be recommended. Homelessness may be a factor and should there be no grounds for detention the ASW should assist in temporary placement. Corroborate as much of the personal details with other informants, family, probation officers, relevant carers and psychiatric teams.

- Should there be no evidence of mental illness or suicide risk a personality disorder should be considered or malingering to avoid prosecution. It is advisable to always discuss the situation with a senior colleague before discharging any patient home off a section 136. Some hospitals insist that only a section 12 approved doctor may recommend this course of action.

- Sedation to minimize any immediate threat of violence may be administered under common law. The initial assessment may be impossible because of the threat of violence and the patient must be 'made safe' first. Make detailed notes documenting the times of any incidents, injuries and medication given. Discuss the level of security needed for admission to be safe (locked ward, open ward, forensic unit). Ensure the ward has adequate staff to supervise such a patient and anticipate problems that may arise. Clarify pass status and ensure that sufficient medication is written up in case an emergency arises or p.r.n. medication be required. Document a clear management plan. If at all possible when the diagnosis is uncertain (section 2) assess patient without medication unless this would add to the risk of violence or self-harm (see p. 25).

THE UNRESPONSIVE PATIENT

Symptoms and clinical features

Stupor is defined as mutism and akinesis: patient appears alert because of eye movements but is unable to initiate speech or action

Clouding of consciousness

Speech usually absent (minimal)

Eyes move as if awake and may follow an object; if closed may resist passive eye opening

Diminished attention span for environmental stimuli

If speech intact, amnesia for personal historical details and identity suggests psychogenic amnesia or fugue state or multiple personality disorder

Anxiety symptoms usually absent

Poor memory of events during stupor

Stable respiration, pulse and blood pressure

No neurological signs: look for signs of head injury, pupillary reaction to light, pupillary symmetry, corneal reflex intact; look for focal signs, localizing cranial nerve lesions, fluctuating conscious level, neck stiffness. Consider the possibility of conversion symptoms if neurological examination and investigations are normal (lumbar puncture, MRI, EEG, glucose, urea and electrolytes, thyroid function tests, liver function tests, follicle-stimulating hormone (FSH), luteinizing hormone (LH), adrenocorticotrophic hormone (ACTH), cortisol, paracetamol, aspirin, alcohol)

Differential diagnosis

Psychiatric

- Schizophrenia: catatonic states, parkinsonian state, neuroleptic malignant syndrome
- Affective psychoses: psychomotor retardation, manic or depressive stupor
- Dissociative states: fugue, psychogenic amnesia, multiple personality disorder
- Malingering/Munchausen syndrome

Organic

- Delirium: consider all the causes paying special attention to closed head injury, post-ictal, electrolyte or endocrine imbalance, space-occupying CNS lesion
- Organic brain disorders: encephalitis or meningitis
- Cerebrovascular accidents: especially bilateral events
- Drug-induced states: phencyclidine (PCP), 'crack', solvents

IMMEDIATE MANAGEMENT

- Ensure that there is no evidence of a life-threatening acute brain syndrome. Exclude the possibility of drug-induced state, neuroleptic malignant syndrome or suicide attempt. Ensure that temperature, cardiovascular, respiratory and neurological observations are stable.

- Take samples for plasma glucose and chemistry as well as for full blood count and endocrine studies; urine dipsticks for blood, ketones and protein; urinary drug screen; immediately check for plasma glucose using glucose dipsticks. If evidence of muscular rigidity obtain a plasma creatinine phosphokinase (CPK).

- Do a full neurological examination including fundi, reflexes and pupillary size and reaction to light; look for parkinsonian symptoms (drug induced); muscular rigidity, labile temperature and blood pressure, raised CPK, raised white count, myoglobinuria and delirium suggest neuroleptic malignant syndrome.

- Obtain an urgent neurological opinion and obtain an MRI scan and EEG, chest X-ray and ECG if indicated clinically.

- Use Glasgow Coma Scale to score degree of impairment of consciousness.

- Examine any past records and obtain informant history; those with psychogenic stupor, amnesia or fugue states often have no personal details or contacts through which to corroborate their account. Verify suicide risk factors, past history of major mental illness and effective treatments as well as recent contact with services.

- If a diagnosis of psychogenic stupor is favoured consider adequate physical care while symptoms are so disabling: e.g. pressure sores, hydration, concomitant physical illness, urinary retention.

- Abreaction and hypnosis may be part of subsequent plan but if immobility is life-threatening and major affective psychosis or catatonia has not been excluded, ECT should be considered as an emergency.

- Consider legal status of patient and whether best managed on medical or psychiatric ward. Common law allows emergency treatment. If evidence of mental illness or suicide risk assess for formal admission for treatment.

THE SEXUALLY DISINHIBITED PATIENT

Sexually disinhibited behaviour may be a manifestation of psychiatric disorder, organic disease or personality organization; it may be goal directed or disorganized; behaviours which would be acceptable privately may be displayed in a public place. The police may become involved if a public offence is committed.

Symptoms and clinical signs

Exposure of genitals: erect penis suggests aggression, flaccid penis suggests inadequacy

Masturbation in public

Genital self-mutilation: guilt, depression, acting on bizarre delusions

Presence of specific sexual dysfunctions or marital problems

Psychosexual history: experience of relationships, successes and failures

Experience of abuse or rape: sexualized behaviour in children or less commonly in adults may indicate sexual trauma

Preferred sexual object: fetishes

Forensic history: violent, sexual and other offences

Clothing: appropriate, reserved, bright colours, self-neglect, exposing body excessively

Conversation: thought disorders, sexual content to delusions, sexually gratifying acts

Physical illness: neurological, endocrine, cardiac, respiratory, neoplasms

Psychotropic and physical medications may impair sexual function and cause euphoria, disinhibition and, especially in the elderly, delirium

Mental state: elation, hallucinations, delusional beliefs, depression, anxiety, gratification from act, aggressive, sadistic personality traits

Approaching other patients or public asking for sexual activity

Sexually explicit conversation

Low intelligence level and cognitive impairment suggest impaired judgement

Differential diagnosis

Psychiatric

- Bipolar disorder: manic episode; depressive episode less common
- Schizophrenia: sexualized behaviour in response to hallucinations or delusions
- Delusional disorder
- Learning difficulties: impaired judgement
- Exhibitionism as an aggressive act; may precede sexual assault or as only means of sexual gratification

Organic

- Delirium
- Dementia (especially Pick's disease)
- Organic mood disorder: manic episode. Frontal lobe dysfunction (tumour, multiple sclerosis, medication)
- Psychoactive substance misuse

IMMEDIATE MANAGEMENT

- Sexual disinhibition may arise in the context of elation when it is goal-directed behaviour or in a disorganized state of delirium or dementia. It may also arise as a clumsy attempt to be intimate when there is impaired judgement either due to dementia or learning difficulties. These situations may arise in A & E, on a ward or in the community. In the latter case either a member of the public or the police are likely to become involved. The police are most likely to be involved if an offence is committed: exhibitionism, sexual assaults, including rape. Those individuals who are clearly suffering from a mood disorder or impaired judgement in the absence of any offence are likely to be guided to hospitals for treatment without charges being pressed.

- The immediate management involves ensuring the safety of the individual and the public. The individual may not be in touch with reality. Obtain as detailed a history as possible taking account of how the elation and a grandiose mental state may affect the information given. Medical, psychiatric and drug history are essential. Informants should be interviewed at every opportunity to establish the time course of the behaviours causing concern. A chronic course suggests dementia. A sudden onset should alert the clinician to the possibility of a physical illness or drug intoxication. Specific details about mood, content of hallucinations and delusional thinking will be important if charges are pressed for any reason. For serious offences, discuss the case with forensic services. A cognitive assessment is essential; if there is any evidence of significantly impaired intelligence, specialist learning difficulty services should be involved. If there is evidence of delirium then this should be treated as a medical emergency. A full physical examination (especially neurological) should be performed. The patient may be in a state of acute distress if assaulted. Admission for treatment of mood disorder or investigation is likely to be necessary.

The Substance Misusing Patient

Patients may present themselves to A & E departments, their GP practice or their families. Alternatively they may be brought to the attention of a psychiatric team by probation officers, social services or the police because of violent behaviour, criminal offences, suicide attempts or obvious distress in public. Patients are often temporary residents and seek drugs out of hours.

Symptoms and clinical signs

PATTERN OF INTERACTION WITH DRUG
Intoxication or withdrawal

Conscious feigning of symptoms to obtain substances with or without self-medication

SPECIFIC PSYCHO-BEHAVIOURAL SIGNS AND SYMPTOMS
Heightened sense of well-being: impulsive, reckless and unpredictable behaviour

Violence: as a consequence of a paranoid psychosis or personality disorder and demands refused. Agitation and overactivity are predisposing factors

Delirium: acute intoxication of any drug but exclude 'ecstasy', which can be fatal; withdrawal symptoms can also present this way

Psychiatric symptoms may be caused by substances but dual diagnoses should be considered: hallucinations, paranoia, anxiety states, depressive symptoms with or without attempts at suicide and deliberate self-harm

Personality disorders: convictions and forensic

history; repeated acts of violence against people or property with no evidence of mental disorder

PHYSICAL SIGNS AND SYMPTOMS

Changes in consciousness level, fever, tachycardia, hypertensive and hypotensive states, cardiac murmurs, needle marks, lymphadenopathy, abscess, pupils dilated or constricted, constipation, diarrhoea

Complications: pneumonia, HIV positive, persistent generalized lymphadenopathy (PGL) and AIDS, hepatitis B positive, fits, respiratory arrest, accidental overdose, septicaemia, infective endocarditis, osteomyelitis, thrombophlebitis, viral infections, dermatological complaints including skin abscess, allergic reactions

Differential diagnosis (dual diagnoses are common)

Psychiatric

- Paranoid schizophrenia
- Bipolar affective disorder: manic episode
- Personality disorder: dissocial
- Munchausen syndrome/malingering: may be related to criminality

Organic

- Delirium: head injury, epileptic automatism, HIV-related dementia, acute confusion
- Drug intoxication: opiate, cocaine, LSD, amphetamines, cannabis, solvents, alcohol

IMMEDIATE MANAGEMENT

- The priority is to exclude coexistent physical illness. If present this needs to be treated alongside any psychiatric symptoms. Problems of acute intoxication and withdrawal include delirium, psychosis, violence. Treatment of withdrawal states may alleviate aggression, anxiety, confusion and psychosis. If there are accompanying behavioural problems or risk to the patient or others because of aggression with or without psychotic symptoms then an admission should be arranged.

- Liaison with specialist drug agencies at the earliest opportunity is essential for the setting of realistic admission objectives and implementation of aftercare plans.

- A contract regarding the availability of all drugs (prescribed and non-prescribed) should be carefully constructed as part of the agreed admission aims. In the absence of an urgent admission each department should have a specific policy regarding the prescribing of drugs of misuse to addicts. *Avoid prescribing unless there are clear signs of withdrawal.* Outpatient referral to a specialist team should be made and the GP should be informed as soon as possible of the contact and of any prescribed drugs. Non-opiates may be successfully used for the symptomatic treatment of opiate withdrawal (propranolol, Lomotil, thioridazine, paracetamol). If already on a reducing regimen and there are clear signs of withdrawal and the decision to prescribe methadone has been taken, then the elixir is preferred. Prescribe only sufficient to avoid a crisis with early involvement of a single agency and keyworker (from primary care or specialist services) to coordinate the total aftercare package. If there are no signs of withdrawal, do not prescribe methadone as an emergency.

- If conscious level is impaired due to intoxication, an admission for observation is necessary to exclude dehydration, respiratory and cardiovascular collapse especially if cocktails (e.g. opiates, solvents or 'crack' cocaine) have been used.

- Deliberate self-harm and suicide: assess suicidal risk. Admission under the Mental Health Act may be necessary if suicidality is due to mental illness.

- Pregnancy: antenatal care may not have been taken up. This opportunity could be used to engage with obstetric services. If withdrawal symptoms are present there is a risk of premature labour and an admission for assessment by paediatrician, obstetrician and specialist drug services should be arranged.

REFERENCES

1   Morgan, H. G. & Priest, P. (1984) Assessment of suicide risk in psychiatric inpatients. *British Journal of Psychiatry* **145**, 467–469. Although about inpatients remains essential reading.

2   Pierce, D. (1984) Suicidal intent and repeated self harm. *Psychological Medicine* **14**, 655–659.

Section III
Psychiatric Wards and Accident and Emergency Departments

ACCIDENT AND EMERGENCY DEPARTMENTS

Sectorization

Geographically defined areas (sectors) have been identified and implemented as the core unit around which psychiatric services are planned and delivered. Each sector has a single team of health-care professionals. This not only facilitates an accurate evaluation of service shortfalls, but also attempts to deliver care to patients within the locality of their own communities. A single named team, named keyworker and named consultant then become responsible for a patient throughout their residence within any one geographical area. This ensures continuity of care for the severely mentally ill requiring longer term rehabilitative care focused on their own unique profile of disabilities. In some localities sector boundaries coincide with social services' boundaries so that care can be more effectively and jointly planned and delivered. Where this arrangement does not exist greater difficulties are encountered when coordinating a comprehensive package of care.[1]

Homelessness

Between 30 and 50% of the homeless population has been identified as suffering from significant mental illness.[2] Such patients may have a history of unstable accommodation because they are unable to coordinate their own affairs or their symptoms are not acceptable to landlords and neighbours and no one attempts to find them accommodation at the appropriate level of support. Because of their intransigence or challenging behaviour such patients may not have a GP. These patients have multiple needs but in view of their geographical instability they are likely to see many doctors and teams without one team remaining in charge of their care regardless of address. Mental health teams concerned with the homeless are being established to address the physical and psychiatric care needs of this population. Such teams should be involved especially on admission as they may be able to offer continuity of care. Hostels also have specific GPs that attend to the physical care of certain patients. Once admitted to hospital, accommodation with appropriate level of support should be pursued and this task should begin on admission by a referral to the sector social work team for a needs assessment. There may also be other social and physical problems. On discharge all problem areas should be addressed in the discharge plan as in this group failure to meet any one need may compromise all other interventions. When assessing homeless patients, enquire in detail about accommodation type, quality, size, length of residence, tenancy. Focus on inadequacies of the accommodation and question whether remedying these shortfalls would avoid or reduce the length of admission. Seek as much information as possible from all sources such as hostel workers, GP, friends, neighbours and informal carers.

Establishing residence

For those with stable addresses and not under the care of any mental health teams their current address should be looked up in the local (hospital-based) directory of catchment areas. Such a directory should be available on each ward, in A & E, and a copy should be available for each duty doctor. A single responsible medical officer (RMO is the consultant) is responsible for each sector. When patients are homeless their most recent address serves as the working address for health and social care arrangements. Where patients are already under the care of a mental health team they remain the team's responsibility until a formal transfer of responsibility has taken place (team to team and RMO to RMO). Establishing residence is vital as soon as contact is made as this determines which agencies and professionals are likely to be involved. If brought to A & E by the police for an offence, the site of offence can serve as the point of residence. This also applies to convicted homeless patients who are awaiting diversion to psychiatric hospitals.

Models of working with accident and emergency staff

'Walk-in' clinic

- Psychiatrist sees all who ask to see a psychiatrist. No screening.
- Senior psychiatric nurse screens all who wish to see a psychiatric professional and refers only those needing to see a psychiatrist.
- Psychiatrist sees all but deals with psychiatric needs only and refers physical care to casualty officer.
- Psychiatrist sees all referrals and deals with physical and psychiatric problems.

Standard accident and emergency

- Screened by casualty triage staff and referred direct to psychiatrist.
- Screened by casualty staff, referred to casualty officer who refers to psychiatrist.
- Managed by casualty officer and referred only if casualty officer wants a specialist opinion.

GP referrals come in by either route and may follow direct referral to psychiatrist, casualty officer or with no direct referral. The latter is likely if there is known to be a 'walk-in' clinic.

Establish clearly what the local procedures are. This avoids endless surprises and frustration with colleagues who may be acting within locally agreed procedural guidelines not known to you. If the procedures are not working because of workload, inappropriate referrals or the needs of certain groups of patients cannot be met within the local model, then instigate change by discussion with senior staff in the A & E and psychiatric departments. It may be time to review the guidelines.

Sources of information

Exploit all sources of accessible information to evaluate accuracy of the history given, previous interventions which have succeeded or failed, and before constructing a treatment plan. Contact previous wards which may have previous notes readily accessible. Some staff members who know your patient well may be on the wards. Old notes should be obtained wherever possible and certainly should be requested if at another hospital. Contact the patient's last consultant and keyworker. If in supported accommodation discuss the options with the housing staff who otherwise may be left to deal with an unworkable treatment plan. If there are social needs identify the allocated social worker or probation services if a forensic history emerges. Always speak with the GP and relatives. They may have the most complete information and be able to list previous interventions and coping strategies for persistent symptoms. Further, any treatment plan must take account of the relatives' and GP's involvement.

Interviewing and safety

Violent assault is not uncommon in psychiatric settings, medical settings and in other public services. In one study 41% of junior doctors had experienced physical violence and 36% had suffered physical injuries; 63% had experienced verbal violence.[3] Ensure that the interview room you are about to use is in sight of other staff, has an alarm button which works and is accessible. Tell other staff you are about to use the interview room. If you anticipate problems do not interview by yourself, however pressed for time you or other staff may be. Ask another staff member to join you. Preferably this should be a psychiatric nurse but in some instances security guards are the only people available. If in doubt interview in an open place whilst making an initial assessment of dangerousness. Never rush into closed interview rooms with people who may be acutely disturbed or whom you suspect of potential malice. If you are frightened then you cannot carry out a sensible assessment so defer until someone can accompany you.

Training and safety

Most organizations should hold training work-shops on how to deal with potentially violent members of the public who may or may not be patients. This should include strategies such as talking down, taking up non-threatening body postures, reminding the potential assailant of your ordinary human qualities such as your name, considering escape techniques and sur-vival strategies should you be taken hostage, raising the alarm and sources of support and information about counselling after such a cri-sis. The use of personal alarms is advisable for men and women; do not walk around isolated hospital sites on your own at night. Ask for an escort from security. Bravado will blind you to the potential dangers. The same advice can be applied to home visits. Do not try to disarm any-one yourself. Ask the individual to give up any weapons and tell them that you are unable to see them until all weapons have been handed in. Ask the police to assist.

WORKING ON PSYCHIATRIC WARDS

Attempted suicide

The Department of Health's *Health of the Nation* targets for suicide prevention are:

1 to reduce the overall rate by 15% by the year 2000;

2 in the severely mentally ill, to reduce the rate by 33% by the year 2000.

Half the people who kill themselves have a current or past psychiatric illness. 'Not all suicides can be prevented even within the best run psychiatric wards'.[4] Inpatients at risk should not be discharged prematurely because of symptomatic improvement alone as this may be misleading and may be followed by relapse on discharge. Alienation of patients can hinder delivery of appropriate levels of care and supervision. In these instances setting boundaries and handing back responsibility to the patient, although a valuable and effective skill when judiciously applied, may be counter-therapeutic. Admission is necessary for those for whom other community-based interventions have failed and/or the risk of completed suicide is too high to justify community management. Changes in the level of supervision, unresolved psychosocial conflicts and non-compliance with medication and failure of follow-up are other factors of relevance in completed suicide after discharge. There are few services that single-handedly can deliver all the components of what is regarded as an optimal package of interventions.

Suicide rates

The annual rates have been increasing in the UK: 48 per 100 000 in 1920–21 to 84 per 100 000 in 1972–73. Although the rates for women have decreased recently, the rates amongst specific groups, for example young Asian women and young black men, have been increasing steadily. Whilst on the ward, 1.3–2.5 patients per 1000 discharges complete suicide.[5] The relative risks of suicide are elevated for young men with schizophrenia (49 times), women with affective psychoses (91 times) and men and women with neuroses (33 times).[6] Social factors such as unemployment, isolation, recent bereavement or separation, being male, elderly or living alone add to the risk irrespective of mental illness. Alcoholism and drug misuse account for up to 29% of inpatient suicides.

Patients will use methods that are readily available and adapt anything in the ward environment: overdoses of concealed tablets, drowning in baths, hanging, self-cutting, jumping off high buildings and out of windows. Setting fires, although less common, is a possibility; if there is a history of fire-setting ensure materials to start a fire are removed. On admission ensure all potential weapons (razor blades, belts, etc.) are given up.

Precautions and observation policy

The ward environment should be carefully planned so as to avoid the high-risk and observation rooms being placed near to opening windows and staircases. Good observational access is essential without being too intrusive. A calm ward atmosphere is necessary as admission onto an acutely disturbed ward will not enable a distressed patient to settle and indeed will distract staff from providing optimal care to each patient. Well-kept, decorated open spaces, low comfortable seats and well-lit wards will encourage patients to stay voluntarily and enable them to feel contained and safe.

On admission assess suicide risk carefully, and make explicit your concerns to the patient, relatives and staff. Ensure that the level of support and supervision during the early stage of admission takes account of the risk factors (and that the keyworker has not yet established a rapport with the patient). Document the level of observation and communicate it verbally to the key-worker. Each unit has specific observation policies. Ensure that both you and the key-worker have the same understanding of the terms 'special' observations and 'continuous' observation. Set the frequency of visual and interpersonal vigilance as well as the time of commencement and review these levels of observation in light of nursing reports. Anticipate reasons why the level of observation may need to be increased or decreased earlier. Clearly state which changes to the treatment plan can be sanctioned without you reassessing the patient. Set a time at which the plan, including an assessment of risk, will be reviewed in light of the immediately preceding assessment period.

At a managerial level there should be adequate staffing numbers to ensure that adequate supervision and support can be delivered. If there is a completed suicide, alert senior staff immediately; do not alter old notes, and immediately make a fresh entry outlining in as much detail as possible the circumstances of the incident and the impressions that the clinical staff had developed regarding risk of suicide when the patient was last seen. Arrange a full multi-disciplinary meeting away from the ward to critically analyse the incident for audit purposes. Examine supportively what procedures and mechanisms were unsuccessful and which additional measures are necessary.

Repeated self-cutting

This can reach epidemic proportions within hospital units. Such self-harm can take the form of superficial cutting with little suicidal intent; deeper cuts that endanger major vessels are not always linked to serious intent; bizarre unpredictable acts of self-mutilation are more common amongst psychotic people and may be fatal if deep cuts are made near to major vessels. Self-cutters tend to be young, female, come from broken homes, have relationship difficulties, may have been subjected to physical and sexual abuse, have few close trusting relationships, may have been subject to early childhood illness, and may have contact with the paramedical professions.

People may cut: impulsively in order to end an intolerable experience; because of severe anxiety, anger or agitation; for a sense of relief that accompanies the cutting and the sight of blood (perhaps mediated by endogenous release of opiates and adrenaline); and where there are distortions of thinking that are depressive in nature and which morbidly rationalize the cutting as the first step in recovery or as a punishment that must be accepted.

Ensure the necessary emergency assessment and treatment of lacerations is carried out before considering the psychiatric management. A behavioural analysis of the sequence of cutting is essential to identify precipitants as well as protective factors. Assess impulsivity, ability to verbalize and explore feelings, distorted cognitions and rationalization, depth of cuts, target areas cut, associated suicidal intent and risk of accidental suicide in the absence of active intent. Make yourself aware of all past acts, motives, social stressors, comorbid states (moods, alcohol misuse), behavioural precursors and coping strategies. Interventions include cognitive therapies, communication work, physical exercise, relaxation techniques, allaying of social stressors and treating depressogenic cognitions as well as other depressive symptoms. Medications include antidepressants, neuroleptics, lithium and carbamazepine. A behavioural contract should be drawn up to effectively link all the strategies.

Management rounds

Models of management rounds

Multidisciplinary management (or ward) rounds have been a common component in the assessment and treatment of psychiatric inpatients. Such rounds include the medical team (consultant, senior registrar, registrar, senior house officer, medical students), nursing staff (primary nurse of each patient along with a senior member of nursing staff, nursing students), social workers (a single one attached to the team or several who visit when their particular patients are being discussed), occupational therapists, psychologists, pharmacists and liaising members of other medical, nursing or social care teams. In the UK the junior doctor traditionally has had the responsibility of making available all the necessary information to facilitate problem-based decision making. This approach is modelled on the role of a junior doctor in the medical profession in the UK generally. Other disciplines either present their own findings or feed back to the junior doctor or another team member. In specialist units only one or two patients may be presented in each round and discussed in great detail, but in standard psychiatric units usually all patients are discussed, with special attention given to newly admitted patients. Patients may or may not all be seen during the round. Such a process has always been put forward as an efficient way of collating all necessary opinions and making joint inter-agency decisions on a once-a-week basis. Although this approach has been the mainstay of inpatient psychiatry in the UK for many years, the majority of patients prefer not to attend or to have an alternative style of round.[7] Also the extent of nurse involvement is sometimes deemed to be insufficient; professional hierarchies are often blamed for limiting the effectiveness of the rounds.[8] The use of management rounds for teaching purposes has also been questioned.[9]

Many clinicians now choose to meet with patients separately as do other members of the team so that the round becomes a decision-making one establishing the framework for care with the primary nurse acting as the patient's advocate. The outcome of the meeting is then discussed with the patient separately and agreed plans are then initiated.

Functions of management rounds

The functions of management rounds include: decision making about medication and psychological therapies; discussion about indications for specific interventions and the impact of any interventions; integration of all the information so far available about the patient's social, psychological and physical well-being; team building, making links with other teams to make or receive face-to-face referrals; and case conferences. Teaching students and mutual exchange of information are other less noticed functions. Meeting and explaining the treatment rationale to family members is another less commonly cited function. Shorter problem-solving management rounds involving the core inpatient treatment team are increasingly common, lending support to the view that treatment decisions should be made more often if a patient's progress is not to be impeded because of the administrative structure of a unit. Daily problem-solving rounds involving junior and some senior staff are becoming increasingly popular in view of the pressure to vacate inpatient beds, the greater complexity of patient problems presented, and the level of disturbance on wards, all reflecting the need to review treatment plans more often in order to optimize progress.

Clinical tasks of the junior doctor

1 Collate all the necessary information from the admission and progress notes and investigations.

2 Do the admission assessments.

3 Liaise with other medical and nursing staff if physical care is necessary.

4 Liaise effectively with other ward staff (all disciplines) so as to ensure that patients receive the appropriate level of care from other disciplines.

5 To plan discharge arrangements in conjunction with all parties likely to be involved in delivering future care.

6 To communicate effectively with GPs.

7 To prepare summaries (admission and discharge).

8 To provide emergency and routine physical care.

9 To record the process and content of the management round and section 117 meetings.

Treatment plans and section 117 meetings

Section 117 of the Mental Health Act, 1983 requires that social services, health-care services and all voluntary organizations involved in care should agree procedures for establishing after-care arrangements.[10] The keyworker coordinates the time and venue of the meeting. Participants include the RMO (consultant), the primary nurse who looks after the patient whilst in hospital, a social worker specializing in mental health work, the GP, the community psychiatric nurse who will be coordinating the community care package, a member of any relevant voluntary organization and the patient and/or a member of their family or an advocate. Each hospital should have agreed procedures for carrying out these meetings and recording the process and outcome. Such planning meetings are essential for those patients who are potentially violent, have forensic histories, have been admitted on a Mental Health Act section or are vulnerable in view of their continuing mental health and social care needs.[11]

MULTIDISCIPLINARY TEAMS

The emergence of diverse models of mental illness and the development of comprehensive treatment packages highlighted that the care of psychiatric patients could only be optimized if the expertise from a number of professional disciplines could be harnessed and effectively applied to supply the best possible care. Community mental health teams have been deemed to be the best way of providing for the specialist needs of certain client groups and also the best way to improve cooperation and collaboration between professionals and agencies.

Types of team (see refs 12, 13 and 14)

- Those that deliver direct care shaped by the needs of clients.
- Those that develop and support other services necessary for clients (e.g. preventative or early intervention services).
- Combinations of the above two approaches depending upon the degree to which respective management and professional structures allow teams to function independently.
- Teams may also be funded largely from one body or have an excess of one profession; the functional success will then be influenced by the dominant group's ideology.

Good team organization requires that there be an operational policy including 'targeted' groups and a mission statement, a definition of the geographical sector and the component team functions, team procedures for receiving and making referrals and discharging clients. Team membership, accountability and supervision structures must be explicit. Team meetings need an agreed structure and decision-making process. Team members' roles need to be specified. Team administration procedures need to be agreed. Individual career and team development should be accommodated and attention given to 'burnout' and 'stress management' amongst team members.

When things go wrong

Dual accountability and influences may lead to role conflict for an individual or several members of a team. Unless the management of such conflict is anticipated poor interpersonal relationships within a team could undermine effective functioning. Fragmentation and burnout are signs of failing team processes and should be identified and dealt with early with a view to the team agreeing to take positive and creative steps to overcome obstacles. Functions within a team may extend beyond or fall short of the roles that any one professional group would regard as acceptable for their profession. The effective management of risk, with dangerous patients for example, needs clear lines of accountability and responsibility, especially where a team usually has much greater flexibility of roles suited to better management of less risky patients. A greater emphasis on operational policies, where key agencies and professionals in a multidisciplinary team have their responsibilities and lines of accountability specified, can prevent such breakdowns of team working.[13,14]

RELATIVES

Families are the main source of support for the majority of the mentally ill. To avoid burnout amongst family members, so that they can continue to be effective in their roles as carers, they need adequate and continuous support, information, timely respite and sufficient time from professionals for consultation. Relatives can provide a vast amount of information for any first presentation; family members have special knowledge of the culture from which an individual comes and they will have their own opinions about the cause of the illness and potential solutions. These should be elicited. The use of a non-blaming approach and developing a working alliance with families as well as the patient is essential.

Several studies have demonstrated lower relapse rates where family interventions are combined with neuroleptic treatment. The concept of high expressed emotion as measured by the Camberwell Family Assessment Interview has been the focus of attention as a very valuable intervention. Other approaches to family working that do not give so much attention to expressed emotion have been shown to be effective and less likely to be misunderstood as blaming the family. Yet both approaches appear to be hampered in practice by the availability of staff with specialist training in these areas.

Involve family members in medication-related decisions: the reasons for prescribing and the adverse and therapeutic effects of medication, but also the limitations of it. Family education, communication and problem solving seem to be important ingredients when combined with case management and work with the individual. This approach is especially important where treatment decisions are controversial, where the illness appears to be resistant to standard treatment approaches or where special circumstances make direct communication with the patient difficult (e.g. hard of hearing, thought-disordered patients, ethnic minorities, uncommunicative patients).

REFERENCES

1   Thornicroft, G. (1995) The case for catchment areas for mental health services. *Psychiatric Bulletin* **19**, 343–345.

2   Scott, J. (1993) Homeless and mental illness. *British Journal of Psychiatry* **162**, 314–324.

3   Schneiden, V. (1993) Violence against doctors. *British Journal of Hospital Medicine* **50**, 6–9.

4   Morgan, H. G. (1992) Suicide prevention. Hazards on the fast lane to community care. *British Journal of Psychiatry* **160**, 149–153.

5   Morgan, G. (1990) Suicide in psychiatric hospitals. In Hawton, K. & Cowen, P. (eds) *Dilemmas and Difficulties in the Management of Psychiatric Patients.* Oxford: Oxford University Press.

6   King, E. (1994) Suicide in the mentally ill. *British Journal of Psychiatry* **165**, 658–663.

7   Foster, H.D., Falkowski, W. & Rollings, J. (1991) A survey of patient attitudes towards inpatient psychiatric ward rounds. *International Journal of Social Psychiatry* **37**, 135–140.

8   Busby, A. & Gilchrist, B. (1992) The role of the nurse in the medical ward round. *Journal of Advanced Nursing* **17**, 339–346.

9   Elliot, D. & Hickam, D. (1993) Attending rounds on inpatient units: differences between medical and non-medical services. *Medical Education* **27**, 503–508.

10 Department of Health & Welsh Office (1990) *Code of Practice. Mental Health Act 1983.* London: HMSO.

11 Royal College of Psychiatrists (1991) *Good Medical Practice in the Aftercare of Potentially Violent or Vulnerable Patients Discharged from Inpatient Psychiatric Treatment.* London: Royal College of Psychiatrists.

12 Ovretveit, J. (1994) Making the team work. *Professional Nurse* **5**(6), 284–288.

13 Ovretveit, J., Temple, H. & Coleman, R. *The Organization and Management of Community Mental Health Teams.* Good Practices in Mental Health, 380–384 Harrow Road, London W9, and Interdisciplinary Association of Mental Health Workers, Department of Educational Studies, University of Surrey, Guildford GU2 5XH.

14 Onyett, S. (1995) Responsibility and accountability in community mental health teams. *Psychiatric Bulletin* **19**, 281–285.

Section IV
The Mental Health Act

Civil sections

Section	Title	Duration	Grounds	Recommendation	Application	Discharge
2	Admission for assessment or assessment followed by treatment	Up to 28 days from admission	Mental disorder of nature or degree which warrants detention in hospital for a limited period *and* detained in interests of own health or safety or that of others	Two doctors, one section 12 approved, within 5 days of each other. Admit within 14 days of last recommendation. One doctor should have previous knowledge of patient. Second doctor must not be from same hospital	Nearest relative ASW (within 14 days of date of application)	RMO Hospital managers Nearest relative giving 72 hours notice but if doctors deem such action to be dangerous this can be barred pending a manager's hearing MHRT: Nearest relative within 28 days Patient within 14 days of detention
3	Admission for treatment	Up to 6 months, renewable after 6 months and then annually	Mental illness, mental impairment, severe mental impairment or psychopathic disorder Of nature or degree which makes it appropriate for him or her to receive medical treatment in hospital Necessary for health or safety of patient and/or protection of others *And* for PD and mental impairment – treatment likely to alleviate or prevent deterioration	As for section 2 One doctor must be approved under section 12(2)	As for section 2 If nearest relative objects, ASW cannot make application but if objection is unreasonable then the ASW may apply to county court to remove the nearest relative	As for section 2 MHRT: Nearest relative within 28 days of RMO barring their right to discharge By patient within 6 months Hospital managers will refer for appeal after 6 months anyway if no previous appeal

Section		Criteria	Duration	Applicant(s)	Nearest relative	Outcome
4	Admission in emergency for assessment	As in section 2 plus urgent necessity	Up to 72 hours from admission on the understanding that section 2 will be organized on admission	Nearest relative or ASW, one doctor, preferably with previous knowledge, within 24 hours of seeing patient	Nearest relative or ASW seen within last 24 hours	After 72 hours, unless second medical recommendation which complies with requirements of section 2
5(4)	Nurse holding power	Appears to be suffering from mental disorder to such a degree that for their health or safety, or that of others, should be immediately restrained from leaving hospital and not practicable to get section 5(2)	6 hours from record of decision in writing	Nurse of prescribed class (RMN in charge of ward)		Ceases on arrival of section 3 doctor. Patient may leave or be discharged unless further detained
5(2)	Detention of patient already in hospital		72 hours (including start of nurse holding power)	Doctor in charge of the case, or his/her nominated deputy (therefore, does not have to be a psychiatrist)		Must be discharged within 72 hours unless further powers of detention are enacted

ASW, approved social worker; MHRT, Mental Health Act Review Tribunal; PD, psychopathic disorder; RMN, registered mental nurse; RMO, responsible medical officer.

IV: THE MENTAL HEALTH ACT

Forensic sections

Title	Diagnostic groups	Grounds	Application	Duration
35 Remand to hospital for a report on the accused's mental condition	Mental illness, psychopathic disorder, mental impairment or severe mental impairment	*Crown Courts* If awaiting trial for an offence punishable by imprisonment (other than murder) *Magistrates' court* If convicted of an offence punishable on summary conviction with imprisonment If charged with such an offence (if the court is satisfied that he or she did the act or made the omission or if he or she has consented to the exercise of the power) If court is satisfied that it would be impracticable to obtain such a report whilst on bail The patient must be admitted within 7 days of the date of remand	Criminal Courts: One medical practitioner approved under section 12(2)	Up to 28 days. Renewable in 28-day periods up to a maximum of 12 weeks. This is not a treatment order and a person remanded cannot be treated against his consent
36 Remand of an accused person to hospital for treatment	Mental illness or severe mental impairment only	*Crown Courts* As above for section 35 Mental illness or severe mental impairment of a nature or degree which makes it appropriate for him or her to be detained in hospital for medical treatment The patient will be admitted within 7 days of the date of remand	Crown Courts only: Two medical practitioners; one must be approved under section 12(2)	As section 35, but can be treated without his or her consent in accordance with Part IV

37 Powers of the courts to order hospital admission or guardianship	As for section 35	*Crown Courts* Any person convicted and punishable by imprisonment (other than murder) *Magistrates' court* Convicted of an offence punishable on summary conviction with imprisonment Charged with such an offence (if the court is satisfied that he or she did the act or made the omission or if he or she has consented to the exercise of the power) That the offender's mental disorder is of a nature or degree which makes it appropriate for him to be detained in hospital for medical treatment In the case of psychopathy or mental impairment such a treatment is likely to alleviate or prevent deterioration in his condition The patient will be admitted within 28 days of the order, and the Region can be expected to specify when the bed will be available	Criminal Courts: As for section 36, but the court must be satisfied on the written or oral evidence of the RMO or the hospital managers that the admission criteria are satisfied	As for section 3: 6 months; can be extended by the RMO by 6 months and thereafter for a year at a time. All patients admitted under a hospital order may appeal to a hospital order. The patient can be discharged by the RMO, hospital managers or MHRT
38 Interim hospital order to assess suitability of making a hospital order	As for section 35	As for section 37 but magistrates' court cannot make such an order on unconvicted persons And that there is reason to suppose that the mental disorder is such that it may be appropriate to make a hospital order	Criminal Courts: As for section 36 but one medical practitioner must be employed by the admitting hospital	Initially up to 12 weeks, followed by periods of 28 days up to a maximum of 6 months. May be converted into a section 37 hospital order by the courts at any stage

Forensic sections – contd

Title	Diagnostic groups	Grounds	Application	Duration
41 Order by higher courts to restrict movements after discharge from hospital (with or without limit of time)	As for section 35	Only for hospital orders The court has to consider the nature of the offence, the antecedents of the offender, the risk of committing further offences if discharged, and the protection of the public from serious harm	Crown Courts only: As for section 36, but one medical practitioner must give oral evidence to the court	Discharge by RMO or managers only with consent of Home Secretary. Discharged by the Home Secretary or MHRT. The RMO must furnish the Home Office with an annual report on the patient
47 Transfer sentenced prisoners to hospital	As for section 35. Home Secretary must be satisfied that transfer of prisoner is expedient considering public interest	As for the criteria for section 37: That the offender's mental disorder is of a nature or degree which makes it appropriate for him to be detained in hospital for medical treatment In the case of psychopathy or mental impairment such a treatment is likely to alleviate or prevent deterioration in his condition The prisoner must be admitted within 14 days of the order	Home Secretary As for section 36	As for section 37
48 Transfer remand prisoners to hospital	As for section 36	As for additional criterion for section 37: That the offender's mental disorder is of a nature or degree which makes it appropriate for him to be detained in hospital for medical treatment The prisoner must be in need of urgent treatment	Home Secretary As for section 36	Until either the accused's case has been dealt with by the court and or he or she has been returned to prison because of recovery from mental disorder
49 Transfer from prison to hospital with restrictions on discharge	As for section 35	As for section 41 but applied to a section 47	Home Secretary As for section 36	The patient can be returned to prison if the Home Secretary requests it. The restriction order ceases to have effect at what would have been the earliest release date, when the section 47/49 becomes in effect a section 37 hospital order

MHRT, Mental Health Act Review Tribunal; RMO, responsible medical officer.

CIVIL AND FORENSIC SECTIONS

These sections of the Act are detailed in the tables on pp. 96–97 and 98–100.

CONSENT TO TREATMENT RULES

The Mental Health Act specifies that medical treatments include care, rehabilitation under medical supervision, physical treatments such as medication and ECT and psychotherapy. Before any treatment can be given, valid consent of the patient must be obtained unless common law or statute law sanctions lawful treatment without consent. For those on a detention order (section 2 or 3 or 37) treatment can be given, for mental disorder only, without consent for the first 3 months of the order. At 3 months the RMO must complete a form 38 (certifying that the patient consents) or seek the completion of form 39 (if the patient refuses treatment) when a second opinion must be sought from the Mental Health Act Commission. Treatment for any physical illness falls outside the remit of the Mental Health Act and must be treated under common law. Blood samples that are necessary to ensure safety when treatment is given under a section of the Act are not covered by the Act but the commission has given guidelines that such precautions (taking blood samples) should be carried out to ensure safety until such a time that a judicial review into the matter is held.

ELECTROCONVULSIVE THERAPY

Where the 3-month period has elapsed from the start of the section and treatment (usually medication) is still necessary or where ECT is considered necessary under any circumstances (on or off section) and the patient does not consent or cannot give informed consent, the second opinion of a Mental Health Act Commissioner (MHAC) is necessary under section 58 of the Act. Only when the MHAC has completed a form 39 can treatment go ahead. In emergencies under section 62 of the Act urgent treatment which is not irreversible or hazardous may be given to save life or to prevent a severe deterioration or to prevent patients behaving violently or being a danger to themselves. Such treatment should be given once and once only in order to be the minimal interference necessary to save life. However, the Commission in practice accepts that should the urgent situation arise again and a second opinion has not yet been secured then treatment under section 62 may be given on more than one occasion but as soon as a crisis is over then ordinary consent to treatment rules apply and a fresh application is necessary for each treatment.

PSYCHOSURGERY AND IMPLANTATION OF SEX HORMONES

These treatments cannot be given unless informed consent is given by the patient *and* an MHAC sanctions that the consent is valid (form

37 part 1) and that treatment is necessary (form 37 part 2). Such treatments are covered under section 57 of the Act. If a patient withholds or withdraws consent at any time treatment cannot be given.

PLAN OF TREATMENT

Under section 59 of the Act, any treatment plan must be specified in whole or part in the patient's case notes and an outline will be included on the certificate. The MHAC may reject all or part of the plan. If the treatment plan is changed and the patient consents then a form 38 needs to be recompleted. If the patient does not consent then an MHAC's opinion and completion of form 39 is necessary to sanction the change in treatment.

THE MENTAL HEALTH ACT COMMISSIONER

When visiting to give a second opinion, the MHAC will need to meet with a nurse, a doctor, and one other professional concerned with the patient's care. He/she will also need to see the section papers with any consent papers, a clear treatment plan (signed by the RMO) and a blank form 39 must be available for them. Having all of this in place will save much time and ensure that the visiting commissioner is fully informed of all the relevant information necessary to come to a decision.

Capacity to Give Consent

In order to have 'capacity' a person must understand what the medical treatment is and why it is proposed in his/her instance. They should understand in general terms the nature of the treatment, its benefits and risks and the risks of not having the treatment. They should be able to exercise choice. 'Capacity' may vary over time and may vary if a person's mental state content interferes with their judgement about the intended treatment and their decision-making ability. The degree of capacity ascribed to an individual is essentially a clinical judgement informed by professional ethics, existing clinical practice and legislation. The definition is likely to change as professional practice, ethics and legal requirements are modified in light of advances in treatment and investigation and in light of specific rulings in instances where all of these professional arenas fail to support a clear course of action and it is deemed necessary. The 'capacity' required to make a decision must reflect the severity of the adverse outcomes if the wrong decision is made. So for a life-threatening illness maximum capacity is required. The presence of mental disorder does not alone indicate abscence of capacity (although the Law Commission are considering this as one indicator) and it is clear that professionals are divided as to the best course of action in specific circumstances of potentially fatal medical illness and refusal of treatment in the absence of mental illness.[1] If in doubt consult with a colleague, and make extensive notes about the content of the decision-making process as well as any final decision. In cases of doubt an application to the High Court should be considered as one approach to secure a declaration that the proposed treatment is lawful.

ADVANCED STATEMENTS

The BMA and the Royal Colleges have produced professional guidelines in the form of a code of practice and explanatory note about advanced statements.[2] The code reflects that advanced statements are legally binding provided the person is competent to make such a statement, is not under duress, has contemplated potential later events and that the statement does not require the doctor to act unlawfully. The implications for psychiatry include the early involvement of patients in the planning process when considering crisis management strategies, for example in anticipation of a deterioration in mental and physical health.

REFERENCES

1   Hardie, T. *et al.* (1995) The emergency treatment of paracetamol overdose: a problem of consent to treatment. *Psychiatric Bulletin* **19**, 7–9.

2   Feenan, D. (1995) Advanced statements about medical treatment. *British Journal of Hospital Medicine* **45**, 107–109.

Section V
Liaison Psychiatry

The daily reality of liaison for many juniors is the assessment of suicidal behaviour. Deliberate self-harm has been of central importance to the development of liaison psychiatry. It has been estimated that there are at least 100 000 hospital referrals per year in England and Wales for attempted suicide. The condition is the commonest reason for acute medical admission in females under 65 years and comes second only to ischaemic heart disease in men. Assessment of suicide risk is discussed on p. 33.

Psychiatrists also have particular expertise in assessing challenging behaviours including hostile, distressed and 'uncooperative' behaviour. As ever, the approach is to be systematic, succinct and respectful in one's opinion (see pp. 27 and 50 for an approach to these groups of patients).

THE LIAISON ASSESSMENT

The referral

1. What for, why now, why worry? Why is this person being brought to my attention now? What are the major concerns about this person? What is the relevant history? Is there a history of challenging behaviours or self-harm? How does this person respond to new professionals or changes in their management?

2. If it is not clear why you are being asked to see the patient, enquire politely of the

referrer what they expect from your visit. The most frequent reasons for referral are:

(a) Assessment of self-harm risk and mental state following overdose or other behaviour.

(b) Assessment of challenging behaviour. This includes hostility, anxiety, distress, withdrawal, refusal to cooperate with staff or treatment and perceived manipulative behaviour. All can usefully be considered within the rubric of abnormal illness behaviour.

(c) The patient has a pre-existing psychiatric illness for which management advice is required.

(d) The patient is thought to have a comorbid or secondary psychiatric disorder on which an opinion is being sought.

(e) There is diagnostic uncertainty.

(f) Somatization or conversion disorder is suspected.

3. Establish the urgency of the referral and how anxious staff are about the patient.

4. Establish whether the patient is expecting your visit – it is generally better if the patient has been primed. If necessary ask politely that the patient be told a psychiatric opinion is being sought.

5. Examine the notes and talk to relevant staff to collect as much first-hand information as you can, particularly about:

(a) Present diagnoses and treatment. What are the associations between this person's physical problems and management and psychiatric morbidity?

(b) Past medical and psychiatric history.

(c) Pre-morbid personality and coping style.

(d) Role of developmental factors and life events.

(e) Somatization: does this person have medically unexplained physical symptoms? Is it appropriate to educate the patient to re-attribute their symptoms?

(f) Attitudes of family/friends/carers/staff towards the episode.

(g) Social factors: what are the sources of external stress and support in this person's life? Consider particularly occupation, relationships, marital/cohabitation, family, social life, money, housing. What is the relevance of gender, ethnic and social class factors?

(h) Organization of care: who currently sees this person, how often and what for? How often do they consult and what do they do?

The interview

1. The interview skills are essentially as for any other psychiatric examination. Try to establish an appropriate level of privacy to interview the patient. See p. 7 for an approach to the mental state examination.

2. Structured interviews are widely available but opinions differ as to their merits (see p. 363).

The report

1. Speak to the key nurse and referring doctor whenever possible and summarize your findings.

2. Write a succinct entry in the medical notes – essentially a formulation (see p. 14 on history taking and note keeping). Cover diagnoses, investigations, suggested physical, psychological and social management, if and when you will be seeing the patient again and who the relevant psychiatric contact point should be. More than one side of paper is probably too much. Further information can be conveyed by letter.

3. Discuss your findings with the patient and agree common ground. Where appropriate discuss also with relatives.

SECONDARY NON-ORGANIC DISORDERS

Definition

Adjustment disorders, anxiety disorders and depressive disorders are the commonest psychological reaction to physical illnesses, both acute and chronic.

Clinical features

See pp. 210 and 231 for a discussion of anxiety and depressive disorders. Adjustment disorders

(ICD-10 F43.2) are periods of subjective distress and emotional disturbance usually interfering with social functioning and performance, arising in a period of adaptation to a significant life change or stressful event. They can take the form of a brief or prolonged depressive reaction, a mixed anxiety and depressive reaction, or occur with predominant disturbance of conduct and emotions, or of conduct alone. Onset is within 1 month of the stressor.

Epidemiology

Adjustment disorders are the commonest psychological reaction to physical illnesses both acute and chronic.

Anxiety disorders have a prevalence of 5–20% among general hospital patients.

Affective disorders can be diagnosed in 20–30% of new medical outpatients. The relationship of psychiatric comorbidity to the outcome of a physical disorder is unclear, some workers suggesting that psychiatric disorder slows recovery from physical illness and some suggesting that those patients with the more serious physical illnesses are more likely to be depressed than those with milder conditions. A proportion of affective disorders persist after discharge especially in those patients with a past psychiatric history.

Basic sciences

A period of psychological readjustment following a physical illness or surgery is a normal and early response but it has been suggested that prolonged and maladaptive adjustment reactions are associated with poorer long-term outcome of the physical condition. Most studies show that the associations of psychological disorders in the physically ill are similar to those in the non-physically ill. Such variables as life events, poor social support, lack of 'mastery' and previous psychiatric history have all been implicated. Although the type and severity of the physical illness is indeed relevant, it is not as important a variable as one might expect.

Differential diagnosis

Appropriate response to illness or mental illness?

Pre-existing or new mental illness?

Some common medical causes of secondary anxiety and depressive disorders:
- Cardiovascular
    Myocardial infarction
    Heart failure
    Dysrhythmias
- Respiratory
    Asthma
    Chronic obstructive airways disease
    Respiratory failure
- Gastrointestinal
    Inflammatory bowel disease
    Peptic ulceration
- Neurological
    Cerebrovascular disorders
    Multiple sclerosis
    Head injury
    Epilepsy
- Endocrine/metabolic
    Electrolyte imbalance
    Hypoglycaemia
    Thyroid disease

Cushing's disease
Addison's disease
Parathyroid disease
Pituitary disorders
- Infective
  HIV with and without AIDS
  Epstein–Barr virus
  Hepatitis
  Syphilis
- Drugs
  Sympathomimetics and their withdrawal
  Sedatives and their withdrawal
  Steroids
  Antihypertensives
  Beta blockers
  Analgesics
  L-dopa

Management

PHYSICAL

Benzodiazepines may be indicated for the short-term mangement of anxiety. If initiated then it should be ensured that they are not continued indefinitely. If the patient meets criteria for a major depressive disorder then an antidepressant should be considered. Appropriate doses should be used bearing in mind the patient's physical condition, the actions and side-effect profile of the drug to be used. See the section on mood disorders on p. 209. Look for prescribed medications that may produce psychological symptoms.

PSYCHOLOGICAL

Simple explanation can go a long way. The indications for specific psychological therapies are discussed on pp. 314–331. Consideration should be given to the need for referral to specific counselling agencies either within the hospital or in the community.

SOCIAL
What is the most appropriate environment in which to manage the patient? Should other agencies be involved to address concerns about accommodation, family, pets, finances?

Prognosis

The majority of adjustment reactions are self-limiting. The naturalistic outcome of mood and anxiety disorders is not as favourable as once thought: up to one-third remain cases at 1 year without effective treatment, emphasizing the need for intervention.

DELIRIUM

Definition

This organic syndrome is the final common pathway for a wide range of pathologies. It is characterized by waxing and waning global disturbances of consciousness and attention, cognition, psychomotor activity, the sleep–wake cycle, and affect.

Clinical features

The rapidly fluctuating course of delirium is often characteristic. There may be lucid intervals. Core symptoms are:

- Impairment of consciousness and attention characteristically in a waxing and waning fashion and with easy distractibility

- Global disturbance of cognition. This may involve disorientation in time and place (rarely person), memory, registration of new material, delusions, illusions, hallucinations and misperceptions and perceptual disturbances in any sensory modality. Visual disturbances, illusions and hallucinations are relatively common
- Psychomotor disturbances: the patient may be overactive (as in delirium tremens) or underactive (as an elderly person with organ failure may sometimes be)
- Emotional disturbances: at times the person may be elated, anxious, depressed, hostile, perplexed or any other emotion
- Neurological features such as dysphasia, dysgraphia, constructional apraxia, abnormalities of gait, tremor, myoclonus, changes in reflexes and muscle tone

Epidemiology

Delirium is associated with many physical illnesses, especially infective and metabolic conditions, any disorders of the central nervous system, substance abuse, prescribed drug taking and end-organ failure. These are also common in certain environments associated with under- or over-stimulation, such as intensive care (30% of patients vs. 10% on medical wards). Overall prevalence estimates among general hospital populations suggest that between one-quarter and one-third of patients have intellectual impairment. By and large, studies do not differentiate between acute, chronic and acute on chronic organic conditions even though the early identification of acute organic states is crucial because of the need to treat the underlying condition and the high associated mortality rates. There is a high risk of delirium in association with increasing age, pre-existing brain disease, substance abuse, burns and HIV-related disorders.

Basic sciences

Diverse aetiologies result in a similar clinical picture. Classically the causes are infective, metabolic, anoxic and endocrine conditions, prescribed drugs, substance abuse, diseases of the central nervous system and end-organ failure. Among the hospitalized elderly the cause may not be established in up to 20%. Male attenders at A & E departments, and inpatients on orthopaedic, surgical and medical wards show a high prevalence of alcohol problems. Many such patients have alcohol-related conditions, but the prevalence of alcohol problems is also high among patients whose current illness is not directly alcohol related, most studies finding that approximately 20–25% of acute hospital admissions are related to alcohol. Thus acute intoxication and withdrawal are common.

Differential diagnosis

The differential diagnoses to be considered are extensive. It is important to focus on easily reversible causes or conditions that will rapidly progress without intervention such as Wernicke's encephalopathy.

CARDIOVASCULAR
Cardiac failure, hypovolaemia or hypoperfusion, myocardial infarction, dysrhythmias, hypertensive encephalopathy

RESPIRATORY
Respiratory failure, anoxia from any cause (remember carbon monoxide poisoning), pulmonary embolus

NEUROLOGICAL
Cerebrovascular accident, space-occupying lesion from any cause especially an intracranial bleed. Multiple sclerosis, Parkinson's disease. Epileptic: post-ictal

METABOLIC/ENDOCRINE
Hypoglycaemia

INFECTIONS
Urinary tract infection, pneumonia, meningitis, encephalitis, atypical infections in the immunocompromised patient, abscess

SUBSTANCE ABUSE
Alcohol: either intoxication or withdrawal. Poisons

PRESCRIBED DRUGS
Either at normal or excess dose. Anticholinergic drugs, antibiotics, analgesics, anti-parkinsonian drugs, anticonvulsants, cardiovascular drugs, psychotropic drugs, sympathomimetics, CNS depressants, cimetidine. Any drug in the elderly should come under suspicion

NUTRITIONAL
Thiamine, B_{12}, folate and niacin deficiencies. Look particularly for Wernicke's encephalopathy: delirium, ophthalmoplegia (lateral gaze palsy), nystagmus, ataxia and peripheral neuropathy

MALIGNANCY
Metastatic or non-metastatic complications

TRAUMA
Head injury, postoperative, burns, major trauma

DEMENTIA
Usually preserved consciousness and insidious onset

OTHER PSYCHIATRIC
Schizophrenia, schizotypal and delusional disorders, mood disorders particularly mania, dissociative disorders, Ganser syndrome, malingering, sensory deprivation

Management

PHYSICAL
Pay particular attention to history and examination. A more thorough cognitive state examination may be necessary. Consider using the Mini Mental State Examination. Also look at current management and investigations: full blood count, urea and electrolytes, liver function tests, calcium, alkaline phosphatase, thyroid function tests, blood gases, blood cultures, lumbar puncture, B_{12}, folate, imaging, psychometric testing. The management then becomes the treatment of the underlying cause.

In the case of agitation opinions differ as to the drug of choice. Many use haloperidol for its relative lack of anticholinergic and hypotensive effects. However it has extrapyramidal side-effects. The lowest effective dose should be used, much lower than for acute psychosis, probably titrating the patient in 500 μg doses by an appropriate route. Some also use benzodiazepines for agitation.

PSYCHOLOGICAL

Generally speaking, staff in intensive-care settings are highly skilled at communicating with delirious patients and know what to do. The aim is to avoid over- or under-stimulation through the use of acceptable lighting levels with clear day/night distinctions and television or other stimuli if appropriate. Clear simple explanations and reassurance for the patient are important.

Prognosis

Often dependent upon prognosis of the underlying physical condition.

SOMATIZATION

Definition

Somatization is best understood as a process rather than a disease and is the most common way for psychiatric disorders to present in non-psychiatric settings as medically unexplained physical symptoms. Somatic symptoms as part of an affective disorder are much more common than somatoform disorder or conversion disorder.

Clinical features

MEDICALLY UNEXPLAINED SOMATIC SYMPTOMS

These are common. Recurrent presentation of medically unexplained physical symptoms with persistent requests for further investigation despite reassurance and negative findings. Comorbid physical disorders might account for the symptoms. The liaison psychiatrist may often be asked to see such patients. There will often be a mood disorder present.

SOMATIZATION DISORDER
Also known in the USA as Briquet's syndrome or Briquet's hysteria this disorder is much less common. It has been criticized as a pejorative diagnosis made by physicians about predominantly female patients they dislike. The sufferer should be <30 years old at onset, have a 'dramatic, complex' medical history and have 25 symptoms in nine groups from a list of 65 in 10 groups covering all systems.

PAIN DISORDER
Formerly called somatoform pain disorder in *Diagnostic and Statistical Manual of Mental Disorders* (3rd edn, revised) (DSM-III-R), the diagnosis was rarely used. However, pain is a frequent complaint. It is unhelpful to distinguish between functional and organic pain. In patients with chronic pain it is more helpful to look for evidence of depression, anxiety, somatization, conversion, malingering and factitious disorder.

DISSOCIATIVE (CONVERSION) DISORDER
Practically this involves a loss or alteration of function suggestive of a physical, usually neurological, condition. Typical examples are paralysis, changes in consciousness, fits, abnormal gait, tremor or aphonia. It may also involve sensory changes such as blindness or anaesthesia.

Epidemiology

Somatic symptoms are very common: 64% of a consecutive series of 94 referrals to a cardiology clinic with chest pain had no underlying physical illness. Certain groups are known to be at particular high risk – those with unexplained somatic symptoms such as irritable bowel, chronic fatigue, facial pain and so on. The range of symptoms is large and somatization occurs in all medical settings. The primary psychiatric diagnosis in most cases is primary affective disorder although a significant majority are suffering from somatoform, dissociative or factitious disorders.

Somatization disorder is reported to have a community prevalence of between 0.03 and 0.4% in the USA. In health-care settings it is reported much more frequently in women (20:1). There are strong associations with other psychiatric disorders, mainly mood, substance abuse and personality disorders. Some research has suggested that first-degree male relatives have increased rates of personality disorder and substance abuse and female relatives have high rates of somatization.

The epidemiology of pain disorder is not clear.

Dissociative (conversion) disorders have been around for a long time as hysteria, yet surprisingly little is known about their epidemiology. They are commoner in women than men. Between 15 and 33% go on to have a physical disorder diagnosed and 33% have a mood disorder at follow-up.

Basic sciences

Dissociative (conversion) disorder in the guise of hysteria was originally assumed to be the manifestation of repressed emotions and feelings. The conversion of anxiety/conflicts to physical symptoms was thought to reduce anxiety about the conflict producing primary gain. The attention of others gives secondary gain. There is no evidence of twin-pair concordance but a slightly higher incidence in first-degree relatives is observed. Abnormal illness behaviour is a useful framework within which to consider the nature of somatization. There is some evidence that life events can precipitate somatization.

Differential diagnosis

PHYSICAL DISORDER
Either alone or with comorbid psychiatric disorder

PSYCHIATRIC DISORDER
Mood disorder, anxiety disorder, adjustment disorder, hypochondriasis, personality disorder, delirium, psychosis

MALINGERING, FACTITIOUS DISORDER (MUNCHAUSEN'S SYNDROME)

Management (see ref. 1)

PHYSICAL
Whether in clinic or inpatient settings, the first step is to review the history, examinations and investigations for evidence of a physical disorder. Otherwise the physical management is of the underlying psychiatric disorder. However, this is unlikely to be achieved before establishing a rapport with the patient.

PSYCHOLOGICAL
It is vitally important to take the patient's complaints seriously. Establish a rapport with the

patient and explain why they are being seen by a psychiatrist. Once a relationship is established it may be helpful to note that the person may be distressed by their symptoms and then ask screening questions about mood and the patient's views on aetiology. The idea is to perform the least number of investigations possible and to then begin to re-attribute the symptoms to allow consideration of psychological factors. Specific psychological therapies have been demonstrated to be effective for some somatic conditions, for example irritable bowel syndrome.

SOCIAL

Attention should be paid to the rewards the patient gains from their illness behaviour, and the response of the person's network, both professional and family. What the person stands to lose by changing should also be considered.

Prognosis

Untreated somatization disorder involves the patient in unnecessary treatments and investigations. Dissociative disorders have a good prognosis if they have an acute onset and the nature of the conflict/life event is clear and resolvable. Poor prognosis is associated with underlying personality disorder and lack of motivation to change.

ONCOLOGY

Psychiatric presentations

- Adjustment disorders
- Bereavement reactions

- Anxiety disorders
- Mood disorders: manic and depressive states
- Suicidality
- Paranoid states
- Delirium
- Substance abuse

Much of the psychiatric morbidity associated with cancer, as with other illnesses, goes unrecognized and untreated. Although exact prevalence data are unavailable it is known that mastectomy, chemotherapy and colostomy are associated with substantial psychiatric morbidity. As in other physical illnesses non-psychotic syndromes such as anxiety and depression predominate. Rates for psychiatric referral and treatment are higher than is usually found in medical and surgical wards, oncology being an area where physicians increasingly recognize the importance of attending to the patient's psychosocial well-being. One area of specific interest is the increasing body of evidence showing that in breast cancer a patient's coping style may influence the outcome of the malignancy. Cognitive behavioural treatments have been designed to optimize patients' coping styles. There are often specialist staff attached to oncology services who can offer excellent support. There is a growing body of evidence that treatment of mood disorders even in terminal care settings can improve quality of life.

THE DYING PATIENT

A further liaison function for the psychiatrist is to work with the terminally ill and the medical and surgical teams that care for them. The diagnosis of terminal illness or malignancy initiates the stages of grieving and coming to terms with the loss of aspirations, health and interpersonal relationships with family and friends. The reactions of patients vary between denial (normal as in the early stages of grief), anxiety states, minor depression and severe depressive states. Those with peripheral cerebral/lung metastases may also suffer organic confusional states. Delirium in the absence of cerebral metastases is a well-known para-neoplastic phenomenon.

The role of the psychiatrist is to facilitate abnormal grief from self-limiting anxiety states (adjustment reactions), facilitate communication between the patient and relatives or friends, assess mood states and consider interventions such as antidepressant medication or cognitive therapy. Problem-solving and anxiety management techniques are of value and enable the patient to plan the remaining days as well as take care of 'unfinished business' in terms of relationships and financial provisions for survivors.

Reactions of the dying patient

- Denial
- Anger
- Bargaining
- Anxiety and depression
- More realistic acceptance

Certain criteria used in the diagnosis of depression need careful evaluation in the terminally ill in view of their occurrence in malignancy. Thus fatigue, lack of energy, poor concentration, preoccupation with death and sleep disturbance, non-recognition and poor treatment of depression in the terminally ill may compromise their ability to arrange final plans for themselves and their families. Rating scales are of value but cut-off score invariably should be higher for population-based instruments. The Hospital Anxiety and Depression Scale (HADS) has been successfully used. The active management should be reviewed frequently and altered if unsuccessful. Interpersonal difficulties, social isolation, poverty, rapidly declining ability to care for self and physical disability all contribute. The treatments (cytotoxics, radiotherapy) themselves are difficult and uncomfortable and uncertainty about the prognosis around treatment cycles will compound the 'understandable' reactions. Explain carefully the purpose of medication, the adverse effect profile, the need to review treatment, and do deliver supportive psychotherapy or specifically target depressive symptoms with cognitive therapy. Be aware of potential interactions of prescribed psychotropic drugs, physical illness in malignancy and cytotoxic drugs. Doses may need to be reduced. Assess suicide risk thoroughly. Much of the work involves supportive psychotherapy.

OBSTETRICS AND GYNAECOLOGY

Psychiatric presentations

- Postpartum blues
- Postnatal depression
- Puerperal psychosis
- Recurrence/exacerbation of pre-existing mental illness

About 50% of women experience postpartum blues with symptoms peaking on the fifth day after birth. Puerperal depression is more serious and prevalence estimates vary between 3 and 16%. Onset occurs within the first postpartum month usually between day 3 and day 14. In the majority of women this will be after they return home and they will often present initially to GPs and health visitors. Education about this condition should be, and usually is, a feature of antenatal care. However, women with this condition rarely report their symptoms to doctors and a simple scale has been developed that could lead to increased detection and earlier intervention. The aetiology of puerperal psychosis is unknown and it occurs following 2.6 per 1000 first births and 1.4 per 1000 in later confinements, with symptoms almost always developing within 2 weeks of delivery. The main preventive strategy lies in the development of liaison links with the obstetric department to identify mothers at risk, for example those with a past history of psychosis, and to offer prompt and efficient services for those who do develop mental illnesses.

Clinical presentation of postnatal mental illness

Puerperal psychosis

Essentially the signs and symptoms can usually be described in accord with existing diagnostic categories. There are special features of postnatal mental illness which should be carefully appraised.

- Content of thoughts related to baby: hostility, anger, fear, evil in baby, death of baby

- Behaviour of mother in relation to baby: overprotective, fulfilling basic care needs, unaware of environmental dangers?
- Prodromal symptoms: irritability, restlessness, fearfulness, sleeplessness, incongruent affect, euphoria
- Apparent clouding of consciousness: presents as confusion, drowsiness, visual hallucinations and illusions
- Paranoid beliefs, persecutory auditory hallucinations (voice of the baby, the devil), schizophreniform and affective symptoms
- Relapse after apparent recovery: more likely in subsequent pregnancies; those with previous history of major mental illness – in 20–50% of cases recurs after childbirth; a fifth go on to have episodes unrelated to pregnancy
- Symptoms can be subtle and careful exploration of any unusual or atypical presentation is needed

Ask about risk factors: single mothers, first birth, complicated pregnancy. Antipsychotics may be necessary. If in any doubt about the safety of the baby admit to a mother and baby unit for assessment of parenting capacity, symptoms and risk to baby. If not admitted and there is a family member to provide daily supervision, ensure frequent review and involve social services, health visitor and a community psychiatric nurse. If there is severely disorganized behaviour due to psychosis and/or medication is insufficient, there is non-compliance or immediate risk to the child, ECT would be indicated to prevent a prolonged separation of mother and child. Otherwise antipsychotics, antidepressants and lithium can be used depending on the symptom profile but these drugs are secreted in breast milk and bottle feeding may therefore be advisable. Trials of oestrogen after birth are currently in progress. Supportive and problem-based psychotherapy may be helpful for the mother after recovery; the father will also need help in dealing with a new baby and his recovering partner and will benefit from information about the illness and the overall management plan. Social treatments include ensuring child care and nurseries for other children and parenting groups.

Postnatal depression

Depressive reactions of lesser severity can usually be managed in the community. Postnatal depression has been shown to have a profound and lasting influence on mother–infant communication, attachment styles and cognitive abilities in later childhood. Preventive work at this stage is increasingly advocated as a worthwhile intervention and is usually delivered by specialist units in liaison with GPs. Risk factors include anxiety in pregnancy, marital dissatisfaction and lack of a confidante, a previous history of pregnancy-unrelated mental illness, previous postnatal depression, family history of major depression especially if a first-degree relative has postnatal depression and problems in the mother's relationship with her own mother. Postnatal depressive states if atypical in presentation can persist if untreated and be insidiously disabling to mother and child. These more chronic states are often difficult to treat. The Edinburgh Postnatal Questionnaire is a useful self-report measure.[2]

Termination

Of women in the post-termination period 10% develop depression or anxiety; psychosis is rare.[3] It is now commonplace to offer brief counselling before termination of pregnancy. This primary preventive strategy has been shown to reduce the likelihood of subsequent psychiatric complications. Psychiatric problems are more common following miscarriage and stillbirth and a well-designed randomized controlled study of prompt bereavement counselling following perinatal deaths backed up by appropriate obstetric support and advice demonstrated that intervention was effective in reducing psychiatric complications at 6 months.

Risk factors: past psychiatric history, poor social support, multiparous, fetal abnormality, belonging to groups that are opposed to termination, younger age groups. Most reactions last less than 3 months. Two-thirds have had previous psychiatric care. Guilt is present in one-third of women before termination and in less than 10% of them at 2 years. There are conflicting estimates of prevalence of chronic cases ranging from one-third at 6 months to 20% at 1–2 years.

HIV INFECTION AND AIDS

Psychiatric presentations

- Adjustment disorders
- Bereavement reactions
- Anxiety disorders
- Mood disorders

- Psychosis
- Delirium
- Substance abuse
- Dementia

Epidemiology

There are both psychological and neuropsychiatric responses to HIV infection and AIDS. Between 11 and 25% of persons with asymptomatic HIV infection have evidence of impairment on neuropsychiatric testing. Psychiatric morbidity has a prevalence of 40–60% among persons with AIDS. Abnormalities on neuropsychological testing occur in 50–60% of AIDS patients. Among hospitalized AIDS patients the prevalence of adjustment or mood disorder is up to 80%. Up to 65% of hospitalized AIDS patients have some degree of cognitive impairment. The prevalence of dementia is 15% and is generally a feature of advanced disease. It is a presenting symptom in only 1–3% of cases.[4]

Management

Immediate management usually focuses on the assessment and management of behavioural problems and neuropsychiatric states (delirium, dementia). HIV services are being established to meet the special needs of HIV-positive patients who have minor anxiety and depressive reactions as well as those developing severe mental illness. Recent evidence indicates that the severely mentally ill (schizophrenia and bipolar disorder) are at high risk of developing HIV because of high-risk sexual behaviour, usually of unprotected sex. Well-integrated services include genito-urinary assessments, medical liaison, counselling services and psychology and psychiatric input aimed at primary, secondary and tertiary prevention. Hospice care for the terminally ill and family support are also necessary components. Some groups (African women, children) need further specialist services that can engage them and provide a service suited to their unique profile of needs.

PSYCHOLOGICAL AND EMOTIONAL PROBLEMS AMONG RELATIVES

- Bereavement reactions
- Adjustment disorders
- Mood disorders

The physical illness of a family member can have serious repercussions for other family members that go beyond practical considerations of financial hardship, the burden of caring for a sick relative and uncertainty about prognosis. Following death of the patient, relatives have to cope with bereavement and readjustment. Following myocardial infarction spouses experience similar levels of psychological distress to the patient. During rehabilitation and when looking after a chronically ill, disabled or dying patient the carer often experiences considerable psychological distress. Among the elderly, when one partner is admitted to hospital, the other may not be able to function alone if the sick person was the primary carer for the couple. The liaison psychiatrist is well placed to suggest staff attend to this area.

The most important strategy involves the provision of adequate and comprehensible information, support and attention given at the appropriate time. Generally a psychiatrist is only involved in this process when a relative becomes acutely disturbed. However, psychiatrists have an important role to play in educating students and staff in this process, a strategy which could also have useful public relations benefits for the liaison psychiatric team.

PSYCHOLOGICAL AND EMOTIONAL PROBLEMS AMONG STAFF

Recent studies among junior hospital doctors have highlighted something that has been known for a long time: working in hospitals is a stressful experience. Levels of anxiety and depression among doctors are high and rates of alcohol and drug abuse and self harm are increased in the medical profession. Over 30% of junior doctors experience significant psychological distress. Rates are even higher among female house officers, 46% of whom were significantly depressed in one study. Within hospitals certain areas are recognized as being particularly stressful such as intensive care units, oncology, paediatric departments and renal dialysis units. Health professionals are generally poor at seeking help for their own mental health problems. Most hospitals have occupational health departments and in some larger hospitals members of the liaison team are involved in the service provided. Opportunities for primary prevention exist in the provision of support and guidance for staff either formally in groups or by easy access to services. At present little training or teaching is provided for medical students on how to recognize symptoms in themselves and the climate does not exist in which sufferers feel comfortable to admit their symptoms and seek help. There is a national counselling service for sick doctors. Local initiatives depend on the occupational health service and acceptance of the psychiatrist and role of the liaison team.

REFERENCES

1   Creed, F., Mayou, R. & Hopkins, A. (eds) (1992) *Medical Symptoms Not Explained by Organic Disease*. London: Gaskell.

2   Cox, J. L, Holden, J. M, Sagovsky, R., Zolese, G. & Blacker, C. (1987) Detection of postnatal depression: development of a 10 item Edinburgh Postnatal Depression Scale. *British Journal of Psychiatry* **160**, 742–749.

3   Zolese (1992) Psychological consequences of therapeutic abortion. *British Journal of Psychiatry*.

4   Everall, I. P. (1995) Neuropsychiatric aspects of HIV infection. *Journal of Neurology, Neurosurgery and Psychiatry* **58**, 399–402.

Section VI
Working in the
Community

COMMUNITY CARE LEGISLATION

The white paper *Caring for People* (1989) set out the policy, while the NHS Community Care Act, 1990 set out the legal framework. Acts of Parliament under which community care services are defined for the purposes of the NHS and Community Care Act are listed below.

National Assistance Act, 1948. Part III section 21(1) as amended by the NHS and Community Care Act states that: 'It shall be the duty of every local authority to provide for persons who, by reason of age, illness, disability or any other circumstances are in need of care and attention which is not otherwise available to them.'

Health Services and Public Health Act, 1968. Section 45(1) of this Act gives local authorities powers to make arrangements to promote the welfare of old people.

National Health Service Act, 1977. Schedule 8, para 3(1) states that every local authority should provide adequate help for households where a person is 'suffering from illness, lying in, an expectant mother, aged, handicapped...' Also gives powers to local authorities to provide services for people who are physically or mentally ill such as day services.

Mental Health Act, 1983. Section 117 imposes a duty of aftercare for certain patients by health authorities and social services. The Care Programme Approach (1991) extends that to all persons in contact with secondary care services. Supervised discharges apply to some persons who have been detained in hospital under the Mental Health Act.

Agencies to involve when planning a service

- Users and carers
- Mental health services
- Social services
- Independent providers
- Voluntary sector agencies
- Primary health care
- Housing departments
- Criminal justice system

COMPONENTS OF A COMPREHENSIVE LOCAL SERVICE

A typical range of service settings for adults is described below.[1]

	Acute/emergency care	Rehabilitation/continuing care
Home-based	Intensive home support Emergency duty teams Sector teams	Domiciliary services Keyworkers Care management
Day care	Day hospitals	Drop-in centres Support groups Employment schemes Day care
Residential	Crisis accommodation Acute units Local secure units	Ordinary housing support Unstaffed group homes Adult placement schemes Residential care homes Mental nursing homes 24-hour NHS accommodation Medium-secure units High-security units

THE CARE PROGRAMME APPROACH (CPA)

The CPA involves a number of elements:

- All persons referred to secondary services
- Systematic *assessment* of health and social care needs
- An agreed *care plan*
- Allocation of a *keyworker*
- Regular *review* of progress
- A *tiered* approach reflecting level of need and service involvement
- A CPA *register*

Relationships between CPA and other legislation and guidance (see ref. 2)

Legislation/guidance	Target group
CPA	All people accepted by specialist psychiatric services
Care management	People on CPA with related social care needs
Supervision register	People on CPA with severe mental illness and who may be a serious risk to self or others
Section 117 aftercare	People discharged after admission under sections 3, 37, 47, 48 of Mental Health Act. CPA also applies. Supervision register may apply
Guardianship	People placed on Guardianship order under MHA. CPA applies. Section 117 and supervision register may apply
Supervised discharge	Some people who have been detained under MHA whilst in hospital. All subject to section 117 and CPA. Many will be on supervision register

SECTORIZATION

Of psychiatric services in the UK more than 80% are sectorized. Ideal population size is less than 50 000 depending on needs, demographics and services. Boundaries may be determined by GP practice, electoral ward, health or local authority borders. Attempts are now being made to ensure that all agencies have co-terminus boundaries. Mental health services must integrate with other local services and agencies.

NEEDS ASSESSMENT (see refs 3 and 4)

Need is the concept that provides a link between a problem and an intervention for that problem. It is a measure of the problem and can be individual or population based. For an individual it can be rated by the patient, the carer or the health professional and involves a direct assessment of an individual's health. In the individual setting a need is only said to exist if there is a problem for which there is an available and accepted intervention. However, where disability exists there may be problem areas for which there are no known or readily available interventions; heated debate often serves to highlight that a patient's perception of need may not be that of the professionals. For professionals, needs assessment attempts to individualize care in a systematic way and also enables the amount of health or illness to be measured in intervention terms. Needs assessment schedules attempt to include questions about areas of need in the population for which the questionnaire was designed. It is unlikely that all populations will have the same profile of needs although a core of needs (housing, benefits, physical health, etc.) is likely to be common to all populations. An aggregate of these individual assessments can give a broader picture of population needs but this process is costly in terms of time and manpower. Other ways to define need have included population-based studies using proxy measures of need as indicators of health or illness at a population level. These include medical information systems, social deprivation indices, service utilization and consumer/public opinion. Clinical care delivery invariably is limited by resources and needs assessments serve as one way of monitoring resource utilization.

DOMICILIARY VISITS

- Do be clear why you are being asked to see the patient at home: Mental Heath Act assessment, diagnostic uncertainty
- Do get as much background information as possible about current presentation and past history
- Do find out who else will be going
- Do say where you are going and who you will notify on your return
- Do take a mobile phone
- Do provide the referrer with verbal feedback at the time
- Do observe usual rules about personal safety in the person's home
- Do not visit alone if at all concerned

- Do take appropriate backup
- Do not overreact

PRIMARY CARE PSYCHIATRY

Pathways to care

Of mental health problems 95% are managed exclusively in primary care. At any one time, the average GP with 2000 patients has 300 with a diagnosed common mental disorder such as depression and anxiety. She or he will have around 10–15 patients with long-term psychotic mental illness on average.

Goldberg and Huxley's[5] five levels and four filters on the pathways to psychiatric care are described below.

Setting	Period prevalence (n/1000 at risk/year)
Level 1 The community	260–315
1st filter The decision to consult -	
Level 2 Total primary care morbidity	230
2nd filter GP recognition -	
Level 3 Conspicuous morbidity	101.5
3rd filter The decision to refer -	
Level 4 Mental illness services	20.8
4th filter Admission to psychiatric beds - - - - - - - - - - - - - - - - -	
Level 5 Psychiatric inpatients	3.8–6.7

Models of primary care liaison

- Conventional outpatient clinic
- Informal meetings

- Shifted outpatients
- Consultation model
- Consultation–liaison model
- Collaborative model

Outpatient referral is the traditional route for obtaining a psychiatric opinion. GPs are clear what they want from such a service.

General practitioner requirements from outpatient services (see ref. 6)

- Rapid assessment
- Shorter referral–appointment interval
- Better communication
- Clear management guidelines
- Statement of objectives of treatment
- Predicted response, complications and side-effects
- Six-monthly review plans for chronic patients
- Clearly stated role of GP and specialist in treatment
- Clarification of prescribing responsibilities
- Information booklets of therapies available

Over the last 25 years more and more psychiatrists have established attachments to primary care settings and a variety of liaison models have emerged. The 'shifted outpatients' is the most simple and common arrangement. The psychiatrist conducts their usual outpatient clinic except that it takes place in a surgery. He or she can offer assessment, crisis intervention and 'hands on' management in the surgery. Patients often prefer being seen in a primary care setting and supervision of trainees is relatively easy. However, no research has been conducted to see if this method helps the primary heath-care team improve their own management skills. A major problem is providing this kind of service to all the practices in a sector. According to the 'consultation model' the psychiatrist advises the GP about management at regular intervals and also sees patients in primary care if required. In the 'consultation–liaison' model the psychiatrist attends practice meetings to discuss management problems with the primary health-care team. He or she may then see the patient accompanied by the GP or other member of the primary health-care team or practice-attached community psychiatric nurse. More patients can be discussed in this way and there is better GP/psychiatrist contact. The collaborative approach is an extension of this model of working reflecting the increasing power of the GP in a primary care-led NHS.

Management: a framework for consultation–liaison

- The referral: consider 'What for, why now, why worry, why change?'
- Diagnoses and personality
- Physical factors
- Somatization
- Psychological factors
- Social factors
- Level of functioning
- Medication
- Organization of care and network involved

The primary concern of the secondary care team is persons with severe mental illness. The majority of persons with depression and anxiety can be managed exclusively in primary care. The psychiatrist has a role to support the primary health-care team in looking after this large group.

In addition to the patient-specific help suggested above, it might also be helpful to think about the practice's strategy for identifying patients with chronic anxiety and depression. A number of simple screening instruments exist that can facilitate this process. Above all, the main aim is to support the primary health-care team in their management of difficult cases by reviewing what the issues are, what has been tried so far and what other possibilities there are. This approach can be supplemented with teaching and educational materials for the primary health-care team.

Primary care of persons with psychotic mental illness

- Clear lines of communication
- Clarity about responsibility
- Named keyworker
- Regular review

GPs are responsible under their terms of service for patients registered with them. The mental health team has responsibilities for persons in contact with services under the CPA. Some favour shared care. Above all clear lines of communication are necessary.

GP fundholding

Since April 1992 GP fundholders have been able to purchase community services including outpatient and community mental health services. Fundholders may wish to stipulate that the patient's GP is involved in care planning meetings, that the practice receives copies of aftercare plans within a specific time-frame and that the keyworker should be in regular contact with the practice.

REFERENCES

1   Department of Health (1994) *Health of the Nation*, 2nd edn. London: HMSO.

2   Department of Health (1995) *Building Bridges*, Appendix 1.1. London: HMSO.

3   Thornicroft, G., Brewin, C. & Wing, J. (1992) *Measuring Mental Health Needs*. London: Gaskell.

4   Wing, J. (1990) Meeting the needs of people with psychiatric disorders. *Social Psychiatry and Psychiatric Epidemiology* **25**, 2–8.

5   Goldberg, D. & Huxley, P. (1992) *Common Mental Disorders: a Bio-social Model*, pp. 15–30. London: Routledge.

6   Strathdee, G. (1994) Psychiatry and general practice – a psychiatric perspective. In: Pullen, I., Wilkinson, G., Wright, A. & Pereira Gray, D. (eds) *Psychiatry and General Practice Today*, pp. 22–35. London: Royal College of Psychiatrists and Royal College of General Practitioners.

Section VII
Special Topics

RAPE

Definition

'Vaginal penetration of a woman or anal penetration of a person of either sex, against their will, without their consent or without regard to obtaining their consent.' Rapists are rarely mentally ill and are usually young men with little sexual experience, personality disorders, previous convictions or other antisocial behaviour.

Although rape is usually a heterosexual act (other than in institutions, such as prisons), male homosexual rape is being reported more often in the UK with several recent cases receiving widespread publicity. In the UK women remain the more common victims. Yet there is evidence from the USA that male rape accounts for up to 10% of reported cases. Amongst women, in one-third of cases rape is committed by someone familiar to the victim. One-fifth of rape victims are gang-raped. Rape is more commonly carried out by young men (over half of assailants are under 25) and over two-thirds are unskilled workers or unemployed. Younger victims are common, especially in gang-rape where teenage victims are not uncommon. Violence accompanies rape in 80% of cases, occurring more often with older women and in gangs. A weapon may have been used to threaten the victim into submission. Although rape usually refers to vaginal intercourse other sexual acts, often humiliating ones, such as anal sex, fellatio, fondling, defecation and urination may be involved.[1]

Meanings of sexual assault

- Power and control
- Expression of aggression and hate

- Male bravado in group rape
- The sexual experience

Reactions in the victim

- Immediate severe fear of threat to life
- Depersonalization
- Adjustment reactions: anxiety, depression – accompanied by intense shame and guilt, suicidal thoughts, self-harm, or self-mutilation, anger and alcohol or substance misuse
- Post-traumatic stress disorder
- Marital/relationship difficulties
- Sexual dysfunction
- Loss of job and income

Management

Provide a quiet comfortable room with a female member of staff. Tolerate anger and disorganized behaviour; allow time to express feelings; ensure any examination of injuries is carried out by an appropriately trained female gynaecologist with specialist forensic knowledge. Involve the police after full discussion (at victim's pace) and once the acute distress has settled. A police surgeon could carry out a detailed interview and also the physical examination if necessary. Avoid bathing until all specimens have been collected. Acute psychiatric states or severe distress may necessitate admission or short-term sedative medication. Contact with a trusted friend, 'rape crisis' organizations and ongoing support and psychotherapy should be encouraged; alternative temporary accommodation is sometimes desirable, hence social needs should be thoroughly assessed.

CHILD SEXUAL ABUSE

Definition

'The involvement of dependant, developmentally immature children and adolescents in sexual activities they do not truly comprehend, to which they are unable to give informed consent; or which violate social taboos or family roles.'[1]

The acts of abuse can involve sexual gratification by exposing children to watching sexual acts or involving them in an act. Reports to date include oral, anal, genital intercourse and rape. Ritualistic and sadistic practices have been described. The incidence and prevalence data are not reliable although some studies indicate that 10% of the adult population admit to sexually abusive experiences as children. The younger the child the less likely that they can verbalize their experience and the more likely that a change in behaviour will be the main indication. If family members are involved or threats have been made, feelings of shame, guilt and a fear of damaging others may delay disclosure.

Disclosure triggers

- Child's report
- Changes in behaviour
- Physical symptoms (vaginal sores, discharge, bleeding, anal bleeding and perineal tears) and injuries

- Sexually precocious behaviour and play inconsistent with the child's age; sexual preoccupations
- Allegation by parent, family member, school teacher, doctor
- Change in performance at school
- Depression
- Severe anxiety symptoms
- Acting out, deliberate self-harm, suicidality
- Anorexia
- Drug and alcohol misuse
- Prostitution

Risk factors

- Parents or carers have had abusive experiences
- Previous abusive experience
- Other types of abuse (emotional, non-accidental injury)
- Parental discord including sexual and marital difficulties
- Alcohol or drug misuse by parent or carer
- Perpetrator has a history of paedophiliac or sexual offences

Assessment

Assessment should involve an experienced child health professional. The psychiatrist's role (if they have first contact or suspicions) is in assessing risk factors, parental mental state, family dynamics, child's developmental state, alerting child health (paediatric and/or child psychiatric) and social services that a joint assessment is necessary. Joint assessments, some of which can take place within child and adolescent services, include an assessment of parenting and child-rearing skills, problem solving within the family and discovering and communicating the wishes of the child. This may be done indirectly through art or other forms of therapy. Child psychologists and psychotherapists have a role to play in understanding the distress, their experience and the child's wishes. Hurried intervention should be avoided as it may cause more harm. It is rare for a child to be removed from parents in an emergency. This may happen if the child discloses the perpetrator and a return home would expose the child to further abuse or maltreatment, or if there is severe emotional and physical damage. For an overview of the management and the essential contents of a medical report, see ref. 2.

THE EEG IN PSYCHIATRY: SHORT NOTES

The EEG is generated in dendrites rather than axons in the cortex and is synchronized in the thalamus. EEG artefacts include blinking, technical or electrode attachment. The signal is very small compared to noise. The normal signal is of the order of 20–40 µV; a signal corresponding to blinking is 100 µV.

ALPHA RHYTHM (8–13 Hz): the main activity, usually posterior and symmetrical. Augmented on right side in right handed. Eye opening causes loss of alpha. Blocked by mental activity and level of arousal. Diurnal variation and menstrual cycle related. Abnormal activity if synchronous and exact temporal relationships between two sides indicates midline pathology. Local one-sided lesion causes reduction in alpha over lesion whilst normal on other side

BETA (>13 Hz): low amplitude, frontal rolandic regions, no changes with eye opening

MU: sharp runs (comb-like), frontal and rolandic regions, infrequent, disappear when opposite arm or leg moved

LAMBDA: occipital, when eyes see a complex pattern each wave follows an eye movement, amplitude depends on illumination

OVERBREATHING: 3 minutes produces transient respiratory alkalosis and symmetrical high-voltage delta activity frontally; this is enhanced by hypoglycaemia

THETA (4-8 Hz) OR DELTA (<4 Hz): scant or absent in healthy volunteers

IMMATURE EEG: frontal theta in young subjects; sharp delta in post-temporal (right > left)

Drowsiness and sleep

STAGE 1: momentary increased alpha and rhythmicity, suddenly disappears leaving a flat trace with low voltage, then reappears. Cycle repeated until sleep

STAGE 2: vertex sharp waves, lambda occipital waves, spindles/sigma rhythm, K complexes (delta rhythm before and after spindles)

STAGE 3: 45 minutes later, mostly delta with some sigma

STAGE 4: continuous delta only

RAPID EYE MOVEMENT (REM) SLEEP: 3–4 episodes a night lasting 20 minutes, 20–25% of total sleep, sawtooth – low voltage and irregular activity as in alert state, large phasic potentials in groups of 3–5. Start in pons then to lateral geniculate nucleus and then to occipital cortex (hence PGO spikes). Rapid eye movements mediated by vestibular nuclei. Reduced muscle tone, more inhibition from reticular system; teeth grinding. Locus coeruleus (noradrenergic pathways) lesions cause reduction in stages 3 and 4 that last about 70–100 minutes; cycle repeats itself every 90 minutes

Sleep phenomena

Usually there is a high-voltage discharge on a background of low-voltage fast activity with vertex sharp waves and runs of sleep spindles (12–14 Hz; mainly frontal) called sigma rhythm. There are also transient lambda waves in the occipital area. Delta activity arises in the deeper stages of sleep. At this stage any stimuli or noise causes a K complex (one or more delta waves followed or preceded by spindles). Deeper sleep is characterized by undisturbed delta activity (irregular and high voltage). Suddenly REM sleep begins: EEG appears alert but subject is unrousable.

EEG and seizures

Generalized epilepsy

Of epileptics 30% have normal inter-ictal EEG; 20% of those with EEG changes develop epilepsy; 100% of those with focal sharp and slow waves develop epilepsy. During the tonic phase there is low-voltage fast activity, a gradual increase in amplitude and decrease in frequency; then groups of spikes arise, separated by slow waves; this marks the onset of the clonic phase. Post-ictal: high-amplitude slow waves with more delta; normalizes over 24–48 hours.

Inter-ictal signs: hard signs include burst of spike and wave (focal or generalized); soft signs include generalized theta/delta. Spikes: high peaks but last < 80 ms. Sharp waves: slower rise and fall than spikes and last > 80 ms.

Petit mal

Spike and wave (3 Hz), bilateral synchrony; focal lesions may produce this frontally.

Cognitive function and epilepsy

The view that people with epilepsy were always cognitively and intellectually impaired was based largely on studies using institutionalized patients with numerous other factors impairing cognitive function. Amongst recent outpatient samples the range of intelligence in patients with epilepsy has been demonstrated to be equal to that of the general population. Other studies that support this position include Rutter's Isle of Wight study, which indicated that cognitive decline was present in children only if there was significant brain damage. In the absence of brain damage the range of intellectual abilities was the same as in the general population. Twin studies indicate that having epilepsy does not reduce the genetic endowment for intelligence unless there is significant brain damage. Only 7% of children who have acute meningitis develop one or more non-febrile seizures at a later date. Only those with persistent neurological sequelae are significantly more likely to have epilepsy.

Epileptic dementia

The concept of epileptic dementia usually reflects intellectual deterioration, memory impairment, impaired judgement, personality deterioration, irritability and rage. It is likely that this description reflects a heterogeneous group of disorders. Heredity, brain damage, psychosocial influences and anticonvulsants are all factors. Interrupted schooling, inter-ictal seizure activity and anticonvulsant toxicity have been identified as contributory. Seizure activity in particular will impair new learning and concentration and, if frequent, will disrupt an educational programme. Most patients can be controlled on a single drug. Phenytoin impairs memory and motor speed even within therapeutic levels. Valproate can impair decision making. Clobazam has been shown to slow mental processing. A reduction in drugs and monotherapy are associated with significant improvement. These effects persist at 6 months and there is no increase in seizure frequency. For those with seizures refractory to treatment the newer anticonvulsants offer an alternative.

Organic lesions and EEG

CEREBRAL TUMOUR: continuous local delta; high voltage 0.5–2 Hz. Temporal mass indicated by a reduction in alpha, low amplitude, slower than on normal side, epileptic spikes/sharp waves with or without delta activity; generally epileptic spikes associated with extracerebral or slow growing intracerebral mass.

Deep lesions lead to bifrontal delta activity (also called monorhythmic sinusoidal delta or frontal intermittent rhythmic delta). Differential diagnoses of bifrontal delta: raised intracranial pressure (ICP), epilepsy, drowsiness in toxic confusional states, in alert patients implies space-occupying lesions, post psychosurgery, thalamic/brainstem lesions, distortion of midline structures.

If a tumour is < 2.5 cm the EEG may be normal. If the focus has an epileptic discharge then lesions < 2.5 cm can be detected. Posterior fossa lesions are less easily detected. Deeply placed lesion may give a distant effect, appearing as if discharge is from surface. The deeper the lesion the more widespread are the changes in the EEG. Rapidly growing tumours cause more abnormality than slow growing; small, slow-growing lesions may be irritative causing a little beta/mu activity. Raised ICP masks local changes; after decompression EEG may then be of value. Tumours as such are silent; delta activity arises from oedema around tumour.

VERTOBROBASILAR ISCHAEMIA: disorganization with a good deal of theta; brief fronto-temporal/temporo-occipital theta asymmetry; theta disappears on eye opening

TRANSIENT GLOBAL AMNESIA: EEG changes within 1–2 days of event (unilateral or bilateral); temporal sharp waves with diffuse background disturbance

MIGRAINE: marked changes, mild between attacks, disorganized background activity and fronto-temporal theta. Tyramine-containing foods exacerbate EEG changes

HEAD INJURY: suppression of normal activity; delta – local or general with or without sharp waves; flattening around haematoma or contusion. In an alpha coma there is a paradoxical increase in delta

SUBACUTE SCLEROSING PANENCEPHALITIS: paroxysms of generalized slow activity every 5–7 seconds; accompanied by jerking of limbs and trunk

HUNTINGTON'S CHOREA: reduction of alpha; sometimes completely disappears leaving flat trace; very low amplitude

ALZHEIMER'S DISEASE: generalized disorganization; loss of alpha intermingled with theta; random high-voltage delta in frontal regions and scattered sharp waves. Sleep EEG shows marked depletion of normal sleep EEG changes

NORMAL AGEING: shows a reduction in alpha, and there is sometimes an increase in beta and theta components

CREUTZFELD-JAKOB DISEASE: loss of background activity; repetitive sharp waves – complexes every 0.5–1 second

CEREBROVASCULAR ACCIDENT: widespread ragged high-voltage activity; very slow delta; if haemorrhage approaches cortex, focal delta activity may be seen. Subdural haematoma or disruption of cortical ribbon leads to flattening of the EEG

PERIODIC LATERALIZED EPILEPTIFORM DIS-CHARGES: follow acute infarction or bleed; there is a change in conscious level, therefore normal hemisphere shows changes also: more theta, less alpha and sleep pattern show prominent spindles and projected bifrontal delta activity. As recovery proceeds, less bifrontal delta and more alpha develops on contralateral side

New anticonvulsants

VIGABATRIN: this is a specific inhibitor of GABA transaminase. Hence the effects of GABA, an inhibitory neurotransmitter, are facilitated. Vigabatrin is used as an adjunctive treatment in patients with partial seizures. It reduces fit frequency by 50% in 50% of patients. Side-effects include drowsiness, dizziness, weight gain, agitation, confusion and rarely psychosis.

LAMOTRIGINE: this drug has been developed as a dihydrofolate reductase inhibitor as it was noticed that several anticonvulsants inhibit folate activity. Its mechanism of action is of interest as it is thought to minimize the release of the neurotransmitter glutamate. Glutamate has been identified as a putative excitotoxin and may have a pathophysiological role in the neurotoxic effect of seizure activity. It has a similar profile of antiepileptic activity as phenytoin and carabamazepine in animal models. It is of value in tonic–clonic seizures, Lennox–Gastaut and partial seizures with or without secondary generalization. It has been evaluated in six crossover trials. About one-quarter of patients experience at least a 50%

reduction in seizure frequency. Valproate inhibits its elimination and requires smaller dose increments on commencing treatment. Its main side-effects are skin rashes, including Stevens–Johnson syndrome.

GABAPENTIN: systemically administered GABA does not cross the blood–brain barrier, hence gabapentin was developed as a GABA analogue that could penetrate neural tissue. Similar range of activity as phenytoin and carbamezepine. There are no interactions reported nor any hepatic metabolism. In about 18–28% of those with refractory seizures there is at least a 50% reduction in seizure frequency. Over 2 years of treatment 70% show some improvement. In 25–50% there is over a 50% reduction in fit frequency. In 20–30% there is no change or a worsening of symptoms.

FELBAMATE: this drug is similar to meprobamate. It is available on a named patient basis only and subject to individual patient registration and to prescription event monitoring. It has a broader spectrum of activity than phenytoin and carbamezepine and is suitable for monotherapy in refractory partial seizures or as adjunct in refractory seizures. It is metabolized by the cytochrome P450 system. The co-prescription of valproate elevates levels of felbamate; phenytoin and carbamezepine induce its metabolism. Felbamate facilitates toxic effects of active metabolites of phenytoin, carabamazepine and valproate.

MRI AND PSYCHIATRY:
SHORT NOTES

Hydrogen nuclei (protons) act as bar magnets when placed within a strong magnetic field; they align themselves along the lines of flux. MRI enables the measurement of the behaviour of protons when influenced by a magnetic field.

Aligned nuclei can be excited by the momentary application of a pulse radiosignal at the right frequency. After the pulse ends, the nuclei realign themselves and in doing so emit a characteristic radiofrequency, the study of which reveals information about the structure (spatial location and tissue density) of the material in which the nuclei are contained. The data are reconstructed into an image. More specifically, the basis is that a hydrogen nucleus is the most common nucleus in biological tissues. Protons spin and their alignment is randomly determined. When spinning protons are placed in a magnetic field they align themselves in the direction of field. The axis of spin is not exactly aligned with that of the magnetic field but circles or 'precesses' a few degrees off that axis. The nuclei of relevance in medical research include ^{13}C, ^{31}P, ^{23}F, ^{17}O and ^{15}N although most standard techniques measure the hydrogen nucleus. A pulse is applied to alter the net magnetic moment by 90°. Energy is absorbed by the system and released after the pulse is removed. Energy is emitted as nuclei return to their previous spin direction. The rate of the energy signal's decay is called relaxation time (RT). Different relaxation times between tissues confer contrast between tissues. The image consists of small cubes or voxels with averaged relaxation times determining their particular colour or shade on a grey scale used to reflect tissue density.

There are three types of signal in MRI:

1. Proton density: the pulse sequence used is the saturation/recovery time obtained by applying a 90° pulse. There is little contrast between soft tissues (grey/white matter) but good contrast between soft tissue and CSF (seen as an outline of the ventricular system).

2. Spin-lattice RT or longitudinal RT (T_1): this represents a return of protons to an axis in line with static magnetic fields. T_1 is the time required for net magnetization after excitation to return to 63% of original value. The relaxation process decays exponentially and varies for different tissues including normal and pathological states. The times are longest in CSF, shorter in grey matter, shorter still in white matter. The RTs of most pathological tissues are longer than those for normal tissue. A low field strength results in greater sensitivity to change but poorer resolution as the voxel size is greater.

3. Spin-spin RT or transverse RT (T_2): the interaction of spinning protons with other spinning nuclei following a 90° pulse interaction results in dephasing of spins. During dephasing, precession loses synchronicity and some nuclei spin more rapidly and some slower than others. T_2 is time required for the signal to decay to 37% of original value. It varies with tissues and depends on field strength.

Types of pulse to improve contrast

Each tissue has its specific T_1 and T_2 value. To improve the contrast between tissues, different types of pulse can be applied.

Inversion recovery

A pulse is applied so that nuclei are at 180° to original direction. They are allowed to relax but in order to measure decay characteristics, a second pulse is applied to maintain 90° alignment.

The time interval between two pulses is called inversion time and can be varied. Varying this enables different degrees of contrast to be obtained. As this is influenced by the T_1 component it is called the T_1 weighted image. It offers the best available distinction between grey and white matter.

Spin echo

A 90° pulse is applied to dephase the spins. Dephasing occurs and is influenced by variable magnetic field strengths resulting in artefacts. Spin echo tries to reduce these artefacts. At a given time (tau) after 90° pulse, a second pulse (180°) is applied. The signal measured at time = twice tau = time to echo (TE). The whole sequence is repeated and the time to repeat is called the repetition time (TR). Although the results have poor anatomical quality they are more sensitive to pathological lesions. The image so produced is called a T_2 weighted image. TE and TR can be varied to improve contrast

Limitations of MRI

Cost and sensitivity to movement artefact, although time-consuming computer-assisted technology is able to average out image densities and 'sharpen' diffuse images.

MRI and psychiatry

A gradient magnet can be used to resonate specific voxels to obtain anatomical localization. A super-conducting magnet gives better resolution. MRI is better for picking up tumours, demyelination and other pathological states. It is less helpful for calcification (plain skull X-ray needed). MRI should be avoided in the first trimester of pregnancy if possible. Metal objects produce a hole in the picture; ensure patients do not have prostheses, aneurysm clips or pacemakers. Posterior fossa lesions are less likely to be missed than with CT and better resolution of the temporal lobe structures is a significant advantage.

MULTIPLE SCLEROSIS: white matter lesions can be detected even in brainstem. The density of the lesions has been shown to be related to the degree of cognitive decline. MRI can also detect asymptomatic lesions. Auditory attention tests correlate with total lesion score

INFARCTS: these can be staged by age; the area of detectable infarct or pathological lesion is smaller than when a single photon emission computerized tomography (SPECT) scanner is used

SCHIZOPHRENIA: medial temporal structural abnormalities (smaller size, less grey matter, smaller hippocampi); shrunken superior temporal gyrus; inconsistent findings of frontal atrophy (also seen on CT). Corpus callosum (thinning in men) and septum pellucidum (fragmentation) changes in early studies

DEMENTIA: periventricular white matter changes are more visible; early hopes to distinguish Alzheimer's disease from vascular types of dementia not fulfilled. Some evidence that the density of white matter changes reflects the degree of impairment

AFFECTIVE DISORDERS: bipolar patients have subcortical white matter lesions; presence associated with more admissions. Those needing ECT demonstrated to have more lesions

EPILEPSY: mesial temporal sclerosis, focal abnormalities detected with higher resolution than with CT. Especially useful for those with epilepsy who develop a psychosis

The Skin and Psychiatry

Pre-existing skin condition

Up to 80% of patients attending a dermatologist have a psychiatric disorder. The social and physical distress caused to patients by a pre-existing skin condition and its comprehensive management may lead to the development of low self-esteem, anxiety and depressive disorders. This is particularly evident amongst teenagers with acne, but of course those with severe psoriasis and eczema usually have to devote much of their daily lives to managing their skin. Unsightly blemishes or eruptions on highly visible areas (hands, face, upper body, genitals) encourage social withdrawal and isolation. Our outward appearance influences the way people react to us socially and hence shapes our sense of self and identity. A change of appearance or a chronic and severely disabling skin condition is experienced as a loss event and parallels can be drawn with bereavement. The daily rituals necessary for some (tar baths, creams, etc.) will occupy them to the exclusion of a job or active social life.

Support groups are helpful but should significant depressive and anxiety symptoms develop then more focused counselling and cognitive behavioural psychotherapy will be required. If biological symptoms of depression arise or the symptoms are severely disabling pharmacological treatments should be considered although their adverse effects could mean that they are unsuitable.

Pre-existing conditions may deteriorate for several reasons. Severe depressive symptoms could prevent a patient from caring for their skin adequately: this includes using creams, baths, attending for assessments as well as maintaining hygiene. Anxiety disorders may be accompanied by excessive scratching preventing healing and also damaging the skin further by lichenification. Scratching may be used to relieve tension or overtly to inflict pain.

No pre-existing skin condition

Stress may itself precipitate certain skin conditions and alleviating stress is known to play a part in managing some skin conditions. Neurodermatitis, pruritus ani, eczema, psoriasis, urticaria, alopecia and rosacea are common examples. Obsessive hand-washing, or taking bleach baths for obsessive cleanliness are examples of behaviour that will not only exacerbate skin conditions but also precipitate them. Skin conditions often accompany ulcerative colitis and rheumatoid arthritis, each of which has recognized emotional associations.

Patients suffering from self-mutilation and deliberate self-harm will have unsightly scars and may require cosmetic surgery, especially if the damage was done to socially exposed skin areas and the patient has recovered and wants a normal lifestyle.

Factitious disorders such as dermatitis artefacta require careful unravelling of the motivation that underlies the behaviour. Seeking illness role, desire for care and love, avoiding other immediate conflicts, deep-seated aggressive personality traits and a sense of injustice may motivate some. Repeated wound breakdown or atypical wounds and healing patterns should alert the clinician.

Psychiatric disorder and preoccupation with skin

Dermatological delusions about infestation, parasitosis and deformity are very difficult to treat unless they are part of a major depressive syndrome. Monosymptomatic delusions, although uncommon, present significant problems of management. Pimozide has traditionally been prescribed but is less often used now because of its potential adverse myocardial effects. Antidepressants and cognitive behavioural strategies are worth pursuing. Such delusions can arise in schizophrenia, paranoid states, organic brain states and alcohol and drug withdrawal. Bizarre reasoning may lead to self-mutilation.

Dysmorphophobia involves an excessive preoccupation with a feature (nose shape, skin blemish, etc.) where there is no apparent abnormality. The most common areas presented are the scalp, face and genital area. Depression and comorbid disorders should be excluded (e.g. social problems, sexually transmitted disease, marital or sexual problems as well as dementia, paranoid psychosis, schizophrenia and visual sensory impairment).

Comorbid psychiatric and skin conditions

Psychotropic drugs can cause skin eruptions. Most commonly lithium treatment can exacerbate pre-existing psoriasis. Light-sensitive dermatitis is common in patients on neuroleptics (especially chlorpromazine) and a sun screen should be advised.

Burns

These present unique problems. Burns may arise from attempts at self-harm, accidental injury or from abusive and assaultative experiences. The psychopathology needing attention will reflect these diverse possibilities. Common to all of these will be bereavement (accompanying disfigurement), disability and depression because of limitations of activity and rehabilitation required if the burns are severe. Self-harm attempts will require simultaneous psychiatric assessment and treatment; traumatic assaultative and abusive experiences will require specialist psychological treatments specific to these problems.

Common strategies

- Specialist support groups exist for most common skin conditions
- Identify comorbid psychopathology and treat at the same time
- Psychological and pharmacological treatments are necessary for specific disorders such as schizophrenia and major depression
- Long-term support and psychotherapy are necessary adjuncts to rehabilitation where the level of disability is severe
- Rationalize the drug regimen
- Consider social care needs for independent living

COURT DIVERSION

Mentally disordered offenders have multiple disabilities that challenge community services. These offenders usually fall between services and are not regarded as an attractive or rewarding group to work with. They often have personality disorders, violence is a potential problem, substance misuse is common and the instability associated with life in and out of prison and crime usually involves periods of homelessness. Some patients do not fall within the remit of forensic psychiatric services as they may not have committed a serious offence and many not always have easily identifiable symptoms of mental illness.

What happened before court diversion?

People who are a threat to the public or likely not to attend court or homeless are usually remanded for reports. This may not be the best way of obtaining reports in a disadvantaged group. The risks are that whilst awaiting a psychiatric assessment in prison, people may commit suicide directly as a result of mental illness; there are often delays in obtaining psychiatric assessments, and other multidisciplinary assessment and treatment is not possible in a prison setting. Even when individuals are identified as ill there will be delays before transfer to hospital; they usually have to wait for a court appearance, there may not be sufficient hospital beds available to take a remanded prisoner, and a bed with the right level of security may not be available (open ward, locked ward, regional secure unit, special hospital). If an individual is not section-able but does suffer a mental illness, when they attend court they will be sentenced or released without any aftercare. The emphasis has been on those who are deemed to require hospital admission. Similarly there are people who are not sectionable and have unmet social care needs that adversely influence their mental states.

Court diversion schemes

The Department of Health Circular 66/90 sought to promote diversion and discontinu-ance mechanisms as a means of ensuring that offenders do not get caught up needlessly in the criminal justice system. Court diversion schemes form the main mechanism by which this philosophy has been instituted. Schemes across the UK vary in their structures, the man-power requirements, the level of training of individuals and in the number of sessions for which they are available. Most schemes include the availability of section 12 approved doctors and nurse specialists with experience of forensic psychiatry. Approved social workers, probation officers, psychologists and ward nurses are less often part of the team but some schemes exist where their valuable contribution is adopted.

The information collated by the court diver-sion scheme staff (psychiatrist or nurse) is pre-sented in court along with any section papers and information about bed availability.[3] The Royal College of Psychiatrists has published guidelines for the aftercare of potentially violent or vulnerable patients discharged from inpatient psychiatric treatment.[4] The Reed report[5] suggests that similar procedures should be invoked in the case of mentally disordered offenders. Thus patients discharged from prison or hospital who have offending histories and a mental illness should have multidisciplinary discharge planning meetings.

Essential information

- Defendant's account of the offence
- Previous psychiatric and forensic history
- Mental state examination specifically addressing whether the mental state warrants detention in hospital and the relationship between the offence and mental state findings at assessment and mental state findings at the time of the offence (these are usually inferred from depositions and witness reports)
- Presence of mental disorder as defined by the Mental Health Act (usually leads to section 35 or 37)
- Defendant's insight into his or her offending behaviour and illness
- Need for treatment and the most appropriate setting
- Dangerousness and absconding risk

Current problems

There will always be people remanded into custody because of their offending history or because of the seriousness of their offence. Some people will develop signs of mental illness when in prison under the stress of being in prison or because of intoxication by or withdrawal from illicit substances. Prison-based diversion schemes are being evaluated. Visiting psychiatrists still do most of the psychiatric assessments in partnership with prison medical officers. Many schemes have no consistent source of funding. Health authorities may not wish to take on a resource-hungry patient with little added finance even though that might mean fewer prison visits by psychiatrists and money saved by the prison service because of fewer and presumably shorter remands. There are practical problems such as arranging transport from court to prison. There remains a lack of beds to receive patients from court and prisons once they are diverted. In some instances individuals have to wait on remand whilst a bed is found.

Court reports: the essentials

Psychiatrist's full name, professional qualifications, place of work, approval for section 12 work status. The interview time, place, duration, others present, all sources of information

The background: the specific question you have been asked to address. Personal, family, social, psychiatric and forensic history. The social and personal history are especially important if a social enquiry report has not been prepared by the probation service. Comment should be made on personality traits including frustration tolerance, relationship experience, any alcohol- or drug-related problems, social effectiveness

An account of the crime as reported by the accused. Fitness to plead: understands nature of charge, can follow proceedings, can instruct counsel, can challenge jurors, know the difference between a plea of guilty and not guilty. The plea: if the plea is guilty, the accused's explanation for events including any sense of guilt or remorse and any mitigating circumstances

The mental state findings: presence of mental illness, impairment or psychopathic disorder? Mental state at the time of the crime; any evidence of *mens rea*, i.e. guilty mind at the time

Recommendation for *medical* treatments; respectful consideration for alternative options

IMPROVING COMPLIANCE AMONG PSYCHIATRIC PATIENTS

Antipsychotic effects of neuroleptics were established in the early 1950s. The effectiveness of prophylactic treatment was established later in the 1970s. Up to 60% of those who stop medication relapse compared to about 16% of those who persist. Studies examining the relapse rates amongst patients who stop indicate that as many as 80% relapse. Non-compliance rates with antipsychotic medication range from 11 to 80%. Almost one-half of patients are reported to be non-compliant within the first year of treatment, and over two-thirds within the first 2 years. It is estimated that almost one-fifth of psychiatric inpatients do not take their drugs regularly despite close supervision. The word compliance reflects an unequal power relationship and allocates blame for a failure of treatment to the patient. The basis of most psychoeducational programmes is that collaboration rather than a demand for compliance will improve treatment adherence. It is established that a failure to take medication does not account for all those who relapse. Family factors (expressed emotion), social stressors, life events, illness and cultural factors also shape the likelihood of relapse.

Strategies to improve effectiveness of drug treatment

- Overview of current information: written and verbal
- Teaching participants about symptoms, and the effects and side-effects of medication
- Increasing participants' awareness of environmental stress and its relationship to relapse
- Preparing patients and relatives for early warning signs of relapse
- Identifying individual strengths and weaknesses and teaching coping strategies
- Increasing collaboration between the patients, their families and staff
- Preparing participants for discharge to enable them to cope on their own
- Encouraging networking among families to lessen isolation and stigma
- Empower patients to take a greater role in their own treatment
- Self-administer medication and evaluate the effect of medication
- Keep the regimen simple
- Tailor to daily rituals
- Provide explicit written instructions
- Implement changes of drug regimens gradually
- Involve the patient in the decision-making process
- Provide warm, positive feedback for compliance and attainment of the therapeutic goals

- Scheduled appointments before patients are discharged
- Shortening the waiting period for appointments
- Using prompts to encourage patients to keep their appointments
- Take an interest in, and have concern about, compliance
- Ensure that the patient and all significant contacts are well informed about medication
- Enlist the help of the patient's family in improving compliance
- Use the minimum amount of medication possible and monitor adverse effects
- Consider alternative regimens using medication with fewer side-effects (clozapine, risperidone)

Substance-misusing patients may require higher neuroleptic doses; disorganized living style adds to uncertainty about timing of medication as does short-term memory impairment after acute intoxication. Those with physical disabilities or those who live far away from the clinic may find it too difficult to attend reviews. Educational interventions that involve the family, daily rituals and regular contact with a health-care professional will help. Amongst patients with poor memories or organizing capacity, dosette boxes are invaluable, allowing patients to know when they have missed a particular dose.

PERSISTENT PSYCHOTIC SYMPTOMS: NON-PHARMACOLOGICAL STRATEGIES

One-quarter to one-third of patients with schizophrenia have hallucinations or delusional beliefs despite adequate doses of antipsychotic medication. Some patients show persistent and disabling negative symptoms such as apathy and social withdrawal but may still sometimes experience hallucinations or paranoia but are reluctant to disclose this or are unable to make sense of and report their experience. Trials of clozapine and risperidone are promising yet some patients show a less than optimal response or refuse consent to these newer drug therapies. Recent attention has focused on psychological approaches amongst the severely mentally ill with persistent hallucinations and delusions.[6,7]

Strategies for persistent hallucinations

BEHAVIOURAL REGIMEN
Social reinforcement
Time out and token punishment
Assertive training to avoid frustration and aggression

ACTIVITY
Exercise to improve confidence, mobility, reduce weight and improve mood symptoms
Posture: lying down, gentle exercise, walking
Leisure: painting, sewing, carpentry

COGNITIVE STRATEGIES
Belief modification: target particular beliefs; induce cognitive dissonance about them, reality test them, offer alternative normalizing explanations
Thought stopping, biofeedback and self-control

SENSORY

Wearing earplugs

Listening to music or watching television

Exposure to hallucinations: repeat content aloud; listen for fixed times in the day only

Arguing with voices

OTHERS

Increasing or reducing social contact

Stimulus control: modulating contact with triggers or cues especially if other urgent tasks needs completion

Self-instruction: anxiety management and rehearsal techniques to talk oneself away from distress

Some patients find temporary relief by the use of complementary treatments which probably reduce arousal and levels of anxiety

RELIGION AND MENTAL HEALTH

Mental illness may present with statements of regret for transgressing religious norms but more often religious content to beliefs is present in psychotic illness. There appears to be a pathoplastic influence in that, more recently, psychotic phenomena are more often expressed with a pseudoscientific explanation, such as transmitters or electronic devices. The decline of religious phenomena amongst delusional explanations may be related to secularization in the West, yet inevitably amongst people who have been exposed to religious teachings there is always the possibility that religious ideology will be deployed by them to explain their experience of illness.

Religious phenomena have also been linked to temporal lobe abnormalities; this is of interest as schizophrenia has, since the development of neuroimaging techniques, been linked to neurodevelopmental abnormalities of the temporal lobe. Hyperreligiosity and a philosophical preoccupation are described as features of the epileptoid personality type also thought to be associated with temporal lobe epilepsy. Temporal lobe damage or developmental abnormality can result in religious delusions; perhaps there is a biological basis to religious thinking. Religious beliefs, as discussed above, act as one influential factor in the appraisal process when illness is experienced. As such, conclusions drawn about an experience inevitably will be consistent with religious ideology. If confession serves as a means of dealing with daily anxieties and ambivalent conflicts about one's morality adequately, then distress is allayed. The confusion surrounding a mental illness can be mitigated by the certainties of religious ritual and belief, which can give an alternative explanation to the meaning of the cosmos compared with a reductionist scientific notion of the problem.

From a western perspective, where religious beliefs are common and beliefs in magic uncommon, patients describing 'magic' may be more easily assigned a label of mental illness than those describing religious beliefs. Societies with standards of normal behaviour often specify times and conditions under which abnormal behaviour can be displayed. These 'rites of reversal' or 'symbolic inversions' are usually displayed at times of festivals or special occasions. However, the behaviours are strictly controlled since their context and timing is arranged in advance. In many non-western societies individuals engaged in interpersonal distress or conflict can display behaviours which to a western-trained psychiatrist may be sufficiently deviant from his or her norms to be identified as a mental illness. Thus in many parts of the world people freely engage in states of possession including hallucinatory states whereby special messages are received from the ancestors or spirits. Possession serves as a culturally sanctioned way of expressing distress, views or wishes not consistent with the rules of society. Ecstatic states and glossolalia can be a part of religious practice, but such practices are not common in the West. These states may be misdiagnosed by a western mental health professional as illness. When a possession state or glossolalia is deemed to be abnormal by those who share a culture with a patient it is more likely to be illness. Thus unusual rituals or states or behaviours that are not familiar to an observer may be consistent with different religious worship but appear as mental illness. Mental health professionals have always to be wary of situations where misdiagnosis may occur. Religious beliefs can be difficult to disentangle from psychopathology where a knowledge of the patient's religious beliefs is absent. Therapists should assess and approach a religious group using its vocabulary and through the social organization of the religious group.

Sharing religion with others of the same ideology secures a supportive culture in which one feels understood and accepted. Religion can be used adaptively or maladaptively and can have a positive or negative impact. Religion is multidimensional and social support is one dimension that is valuable. Religious support systems may compete with statutory services as the preferred option and it may be that for a particular patient they serve a more satisfactory solution; knowing that one can share in the care of others and oneself in a community can give a sense of purpose to an otherwise isolated group of people who are no longer in stable relationships or have lost their loved ones. God can be seen as a protective influence and belief in ultimate salvation can remove the intensity of anxiety surrounding a situation the outcome of which is unclear. Religious leaders are influential and a patient's peers in a religious community may be able to persuade and support a patient in seeking help and engaging in services. Of particular value is the view of a patient's religious leader about beliefs and behaviour in which a potential patient engages. The leader may suggest a complete absence of any abnormality or may point out what discrepancies there are with healthy religious activity hence further improving the reliability with which diagnoses can be made across religious boundaries. If models of health and illness are shared then better understanding of a problem is possible. Where models differ (in the absence of delusional beliefs) then treatment offered may be rejected as it would break religious taboos and threaten the safety and security that religion affords to those in distress.

Religion and mental health: arenas of shared influence

ILLNESS EXPERIENCE AND DEALING WITH DISTRESS

Ways of conceptualizing misfortune: explanations of illness experience

Making sense of events: a punishment or suffering sent by God which is to be accepted

Constructs about help seeking

Prescriptions about dealing with strong emotions such as anger

RITES OF PASSAGE: FAMILY, MARRIAGE, CHILDREN, BIRTH AND DEATH

Adhering to prescribed patterns of marriage: who, when, why and why not

Acceptable family structures, single parenthood

Ways of dealing with family disagreements, distress and social problems

Marriage arrangements; limitations of partner's religion, culture, social class

Pre-marital sex may be acceptable or forbidden

Sexual activity: frequency, prohibitions, special observances and taboos, homosexuality

Children: education, style of reinforcing societal norms

Role of women in society

Ceremonies for birth and death

RELIGIOUS PRACTICE, RITUAL, IDEOLOGY AND ORGANIZATIONS

Emotional support from religious certainty leading to hope and forward planning

Emotional support from one's friends and religious leaders

Work may be seen to be an essential to fulfilment

Pathways to salvation: what acts must be done and in what time-frame

Rules by which one lives. Is state law separate from religious law?

Definitions of deviance reinforced

Prayer and religious ritual: distraction, hope, communication with one's self

A sense of belonging

Functions of religion

- Religion serves as a filter articulating the illness experience in mental disorder
- Religion, metaphors and idioms of distress are used to verbalize the appraisal of illness experience
- Religious content of beliefs in mental illness
- Religion informs help seeking

- Clinically difficulties arise when trying to differentiate between religious fervour, ecstatic states, possession and mental illness
- Religious communities may have their own coping strategies (prayer/confession) – these should be considered in the treatment plan

THE EMERGENCY CROSS-CULTURAL PSYCHIATRIC ASSESSMENT

Communication and cultural distance

These are general guidelines aimed at ensuring safe and sensitive practice and do not represent a recipe of how to do it culture by culture. Before an assessment note the first and preferred language in which the patient communicates. If this is not English find an interpreter. Be aware of your own and the patient's body language. During the initial part of the assessment try to identify idioms of distress and 'emotional' words used by the patient.

Pitfalls in the cross-cultural assessment

Cultural camouflage: mentally ill patients may encourage your perception of not understanding their culture and rationalize their symptoms as being in accord with their culture. Do not dismiss a patient's or relative's complaints if you are persuaded that there is enough evidence of mental illness and the patient needs urgent treatment and home treatment will fail.

You may be under pressure from relatives and friends not to admit or label because of stigma, impact on self-esteem and fear of being 'locked way'. If during a crisis you are unable to address all of the patient's, family's and advocate's concerns arrange a special meeting with them to convey your concerns after the patient is 'safely managed'. Make sure you convey the risks you are taking, the risks you are prepared to take and the risks they are asking you to take. Where there is doubt about the assessment and diagnosis, if all parties are prepared to share the risks, and the patient is not in need of hospitalization, then more creative treatment interventions can be considered in terms of location, type of intervention and personnel involved. The more difficult the decision the more important it is that a proper case conference is held as soon as possible involving all parties.

Be aware that delusional beliefs, religious beliefs and the degree of insight are very difficult to conclusively assess in a different culture.

Terms for ethnic identity do not convey the degree of identification with any specific community, religion or language and should be carefully applied. The limitations of such categories for each patient should be specified.

Identify during the assessment the sense of belonging, family structure, family roles, where the patient fits into these, role expectations in the context of their culture and styles of dealing with distress or conflict. Second- and third-generation children have varying degrees of western identity, views, health beliefs and religious commitment.

Anthropology has shed much light on the limitations of western psychiatry yet it remains a western science in itself. Thus there is always the possibility that value judgements and culturally insensitive practice enter the interaction between patient and health professional.

Do not underestimate the impact of discrimination in the patient's life – this will undermine trust.

Do not miss culturally consistent behaviours that differ in quality or quantity from those that the patient's reference group consider within cultural bounds.

Setting up the assessment

- Know your limits: be aware of your own culture and how your skills may therefore be blunted
- Know the patient's limits: assume nothing about the patient; assess which is the predominant group with which the patient identifies
- Know the family's limits: their language limitations, sense of urgency and crisis and capacity to support the patient should home-based treatment be chosen
- Know the interpreter's limits: meet with them before the assessment; ensure the interpreter is from the same culture, identify sources of difference (e.g. dialect, religion). Agree the method of working together: literal translation of all material, will you use the interpreter to assess the cultural context of complaints, does the patient have any objections to this particular interpreter?
- Identify the most important information you need
- Identify the most important information the patient wants to find out
- Identify the most important information the patient's family and friends want to know

Practice points

- For each of the parties involved in the consultation elicit: first language, place of birth, religion, parental place of birth, self-defined ethnicity, identifications with specific cultural groups

- Define and redefine terms used by you and the patient to ensure a shared understanding of the problem

- Critically ask for clarification about signs or symptoms that seem unusual or simply bizarre: explore the experience and then the meaning of the experience to the patient and his/her family

- Do not be judgemental about patterns of communication or domination of an interview by one family member. This may be their designated role

- Be sensitive to the effect of your actions, the setting, or the referral mode which jeopardizes trust. For example, communicate that total confidentiality will be observed

- Specifically, be sensitive to religious and social taboos within the patient's culture. Similarly, women may prefer to be seen by a woman.

- Do not ask relatives and children to interpret

- Involve independent advocates early; this should be done with the patient's agreement

- You must discuss the findings with an independent person properly familiar with the patient's cultural background. This preferably should be a member of the health professions but many voluntary organizations offer this advocacy role

- If you do not know for certain, do not assume anything about the patient

- Some patients will express explanations of their state that may sound like delusional content: for example in one study explanatory models amongst Indians included sorcery (10%), possession by demons or deities (33%), humoral imbalance (15%), violations of taboo (5%) and external stressors (33%)

Management

This consists of carefully balancing the treatment requirements with the patient's wishes, taking account of cultural distance and that you may be making a decision based on much less information than is usual. This makes it more likely that you will make the wrong decision and requires that you carry out a careful risk assessment. Do not prescribe symptomatically if the diagnosis is unclear. This will lead to false expectations on the part of the patient and may expose them to adverse side-effects that render them less inclined to return or take medication in the future.

If not urgent and there is insufficient time, arrange a further assessment time. This will allow you to think about the patient's presentation, obtain supervision and obtain corroborative information from past records, doctors, social workers and other family members familiar with the cultural context. Let the patient know that you will be making enquiries. They may object.

If urgent and a crisis admission is required avoid medication if possible until further assessment on the ward has taken place. Do not admit under section in the following circumstances: of linguistic isolation or the absence of an interpreter; where the presentation does not make sense and further assessment would be helpful but the patient refuses admission; where there are no immediate indicators of major mental illness or risk of self-harm. If you are sure that there are major signs or symptoms of mental illness and/or a risk of serious self-harm, admit the patient. Discuss the plan with the patient and his or her relatives. Be aware that placing a patient onto an unfamiliar ward environment may exacerbate their mental state and necessitate urgent medication. Be aware that the relatives may be unable to manage the patient on their own despite their best intentions and their wish to take the patient home in accord with his or her wishes.

CULTURE-BOUND SYNDROMES

These are defined as a group of disorders confined to a single culture or area. They are popular examination topics, but usually when such exotic disorders are discovered there is a flurry of case reports indicating the existence of a syndrome in other cultures also; the original pathological interpretation placed on a behaviour or syndrome retrospectively is identified to have arisen out of poor communication and culturally based ethnocentric value judgements by the observer. Such syndromes have a range of symbolic meanings that are not readily translated across cultures and are often embedded in the sociopolitical history of a society. Agoraphobia, parasuicide and anorexia have been described as western culture-bound syndromes of the industrialized nations.[8] Some of these better-known syndromes are listed.

Koro was originally described in Chinese men and is a fear of the penis shrinking into the abdomen. Some men even tie a piece of string around the penis to prevent it disappearing or ask their partner to hold onto it. It is regarded as an anxiety state.

Dhat was originally described amongst Indian men who characteristically complain of loss of semen in the urine. They have multiple aches and report that loss of semen is causing them weakness. It is regarded as an anxiety state but reports indicate that it does respond to antidepressant medication.

Windigo was originally described in North America as a compulsive desire to become a cannibal. This syndrome has since been discredited as an artefact of poor communication and premature assumptions about the behaviour.

Susto is also known as soul loss in Latin America. It is considered to be a depressive state.

Shinkeishitsu is an anxiety stage described amongst Japanese men. It is a syndrome of obsessionality and anxiety symptoms.

Latah consists of automatic stylized imitative behaviour including posturing and the utterance of obscenities immediately after a startle reaction. It seems that the biological basis of this exaggerated startle reaction is common to all cultures but identified and reinforced to have some social and cultural meaning in South East Asia.

It is better not to try and shape the psychiatric presentation to one of these syndromes but rather to specify what aspects of the patient's presentation may be better understood by comparison with these local syndromes, which are likely to undergo change in any case.

POSSESSION STATES

The term 'possession' means many things to the lay public but usually evokes a picture of demonic possession. Such states are reported generally as the experience of a spirit entering and taking control of an individual. Various perspectives deriving from disciplines including sociology, anthropology, theology and psychopathology have enabled a better understanding of possession.[9] Possession states are common universally and are culturally accepted in about 90% of the world's population.[10]

> Demonic possession is characterized by sudden sensory and motor changes (anaesthesia to pain and temperature; feats of enormous strength), sudden alteration of conscious level and an audible (to observers) change in voice. It is this type of possession in which religious ideology plays the greater part although the mechanism may be dissociative according to western theories; specifically there appears to be no objective account of a change in conscious level. Features vary from culture to culture so that the manifestation and resolution of such states are culturally determined in accord with the lay and religious body of knowledge about such phenomena. Indeed a failure of exorcism is regarded in some cultures as evidence of mental illness.
>
> Sociocultural possession states are regarded as culturally sanctioned methods of resolving interpersonal and community distress where other methods of resolution do not exist. Commonly these are cited to occur amongst those who have no culturally appropriate method of protesting; they are common amongst women, for example in cultures where women's status is not regarded as high and where they have placed upon them impossible expectations and obligations (Zar possession states). This type of possession and its treatment are socialized events and serve a function within a society.

Finally possession as a symptom of mental illness is usually manifest as delusional beliefs about being possessed. The illness then would not respond to exorcism.

Psychiatric differential diagnosis

Schizophrenia, affective disorders and schizoaffective states

Brief reactive psychosis

Personality disorders: multiple and borderline types

Organic disorders

Temporal lobe epilepsy

Head injury

Psychoactive substance intoxication

Sensory deprivation and other extreme states of deprivation

Management (see ref. 9)

Possession states require a comprehensive social, psychiatric, biological and cultural assessment. A full psychiatric history, mental state and physical examination are required. It is important to have a thorough neurological assessment because of the possibility of an organic disorder presenting in this way.

- Ritualized trance states (e.g. mediums assuming conscious control of events)
- Suggestibility phenomena (e.g. faith healing, witchcraft, voodoo)
- Dissociative phenomena (include brief psychosis or conversion symptoms)

- Delusional possession as a symptom of a mental illness

The management is the same as for the generic psychiatric disorder diagnosed; notably those with dissociative features benefit from benzodiazepines to contain symptoms (rather than neuroleptics), along with abreaction and psychotherapy aimed at identifying the conflicts. Those with delusional possession require antipsychotic pharmacological and psychotherapeutic (cognitive behavioural) treatments. Traditional culturally sanctioned mechanisms of resolving distress are likely to be unsuccessful if applied to patients who have delusional possession states but may be helpful in those with dissociative disorders.

The difficulty lies in distinguishing the dissociative group from those with suggestibility states. Therefore the assessment of suggestibility, ritualized and dissociative states will require consultation with those having expert knowledge about religious, cultural, spiritual and sociological aspects of possession states. Members of the community to which the patient belongs should be consulted at all stages of the assessment and treatment process.

REFERENCES

1   Bancroft J. (1989) *Human Sexuality and its Problems*. London: Churchill Livingstone.

2   DHSS (1988) *Diagnosis of Child Sexual Abuse: Guidance for Doctors*. London: HMSO.

3   Carson, D. (1985) Doctors in the witness box. *British Journal of Hospital Medicine* **33**, 283–286.

4 Royal College of Psychiatrists (1991) *Good Medical Practice in the Aftercare of Potentially Violent or Vulnerable Patients Discharged from Inpatient Psychiatric Treatment*. London: Royal College of Psychiatrists.

5 Reed, J. (1992) *Review of the Health and Social Services for Mentally Disordered Offenders and Others Requiring Similar Services*. Final Summary Report. London: HMSO.

6 Kingdon, D. & Turkington, D. (1994) *Cognitive Behaviour Therapy of Schizophrenia*. New York: Guilford.

7 Huckle, P. L. & Palia, S. S. (1993) Managing resistant schizophrenia. *British Journal of Hospital Medicine* **50**, 467–471.

8 Helman, C. G. (1990) *Culture, Health and Illness*. Oxford: Butterworth Heinemann.

9 Perera, S., Bhui, K. & Dein, S. (1995) Making sense of possession states. *British Journal of Hospital Medicine* **53**, 582.

10 Ward, C. (1989) Possession and exorcism: psychopathology and psychotherapy in a magico-religious context. In: Ward, C. (ed.) *Altered States of Consciousness and Mental Health*. pp. 125–144. California: Sage.

Section VIII
Specific Conditions

DEMENTIA

Definition

Global deterioration of higher cortical function, manifesting as decline in memory, thinking, orientation, comprehension, language, intellect, personality and behaviour resulting from diffuse organic disease of the cerebral hemispheres or subcortical structures. Usually, but not necessarily, progressive and irreversible. Cognitive decline begins most commonly with a deterioration in short-term memory and immediate recall, and progresses to global intellectual deterioration.

According to the International Classification of Diseases (ICD)-10 the primary requirement for a diagnosis of dementia is 'evidence of a decline in both memory and thinking which is sufficient to impair personal activities of daily living'. The symptoms of dementia must have been present for *at least 6 months* for a diagnosis to be made.

Clinical features

Early signs and symptoms

- Memory impairment for recent events and poor retention of new information: registers information but 5-minute recall impaired, though memory for distant events often preserved
- Reduction in range of interests
- Poverty of thought, perseveration and persecutory beliefs
- Subtle change in personality: may

become irritable or aggressive, with occasional outbursts

- Changes in mood: anxiety and depression, or mood may be labile
- Change in behaviour: restless, distractible, sometimes antisocial (e.g. 'social lapses' such as shoplifting), rigid and stereotyped routines. May be suspicious and possibly physically aggressive and/or violent

Remember that clinical features of dementia are influenced by pre-morbid cognitive/intellectual abilities and personality. Those with high pre-morbid IQ and/or good social skills may be able to compensate for early symptoms.

Late signs and symptoms

- Further memory loss including memory for distant events
- Disorientation especially in time but also in place and, later, person; may lead to wandering
- Self-neglect and deterioration in self-care
- Restlessness especially afternoons and evenings
- Dyspraxias, dysphasias, and agnosias
- Mannerisms and stereotypies including ceaseless pacing
- Incoherence or mutism
- Incontinence of urine and faeces

Epidemiology

The most common psychiatric disorder among the elderly. Estimated prevalence of severe dementia is 3–5% among those aged over 65 years, and 20% among those aged 80 years and over. The estimated annual incidence of severe dementia is 0.5–1.0% among those aged 70–79 years, and 2.0–2.5% among those aged over 80 years.

No consistent sex difference has been identified in the prevalence or incidence of severe dementia.

Mild dementia affects up to 10% of those over 65 years and 25% of those over 80 years.

Basic sciences

Approximately 50% of all dementias are of the *Alzheimer's type* (ICD-10 F00), characterized by cerebral atrophy and enlarged ventricles on CT scan. Pathognomonic histopathological findings are a reduction in the number of neurones, accompanied by senile plaques (with beta-amyloid core), and neurofibrillary tangles (made of paired helical filaments). Cholinergic neurones are particularly affected, with evidence of reduced levels of acetylcholine and choline acetyltransferase. Cerebral changes are most prominent in the hippocampus, locus coeruleus and tempo-parietal and frontal cortex.

The other main type of dementia identified is *vascular dementia* (ICD-10 F01), which includes multi-infarct dementia. In contrast to Alzheimer's disease, which has an insidious onset and progresses steadily over 2 or 3 years, vascular dementia tends to occur in the context of a history of transient ischaemic attacks or cerebrovascular accidents, and has a more 'step-wise' course.

For Alzheimer's disease, main risk factors are a positive family history and advancing age.

Recent research has identified an association between the presence of the gene responsible for apolipoprotein E (*ApoE*) and an increased risk of Alzheimer's disease. Though this association has been found in sporadic (non-familial) cases of Alzheimer's disease, it may be that the *ApoE* gene further increases the risk of Alzheimer's disease among those with a positive family history.

Dementia also occurs commonly among those with a history of severe and/or repeated head injury, such as boxers ('dementia pugilistica').

Differential diagnosis

Organic

- Normal ageing may mimic mild dementia, especially if stressed
- Delirium (acute confusional state) (see p. 198). Likely to be associated with infection, e.g. respiratory tract infection. Supported by evidence of impaired level of consciousness, with lucid intervals and/or diurnal changes in symptom intensity. Delusions and/or hallucinations usually rich in ideas and associations, and devoid of negative affective flavour found in depression. Unlike dementia, symptoms are almost always reversible
- Amnesic syndrome (Korsakoff's syndrome) resulting from alcohol abuse and characterized by severe deficit in short-term memory and confabulation
- Reversible forms of dementia including:

    (i)   Multi-infarct dementia, associated with hypertension and character-

(ii)   ized by focal neurological deficits, stepwise progression, and pseudobulbar signs

(ii)   Normal pressure hydrocephalus, characterized by gait ataxia, incontinence and progressive dementia. May result from trauma, haemorrhage or infection. CSF pressure is normal but ventricles are dilated on CT scan

(iii)   Drug intoxication, commonly iatrogenic: likely candidates are digoxin, benzodiazepines, analgesics and methyldopa

(iv)   Subdural haematoma

(v)   Tumours

(vi)   Metabolic disorders, particularly hypothyroidism

(vii) B_{12} or folate deficiency

(viii)   Hepatic or renal failure

(ix)   Infectious causes, namely tuberculosis, toxoplasmosis, cerebral abscess or neurosyphilis

Psychiatric

Depression must *always* be considered, particularly where history of 'acute' cognitive impairment. Cognitive impairment may be marked, due to severe psychomotor retardation, hence the name 'pseudodementia'. Unlike those with dementia, who may try to deny cognitive decline, elderly patients with depression complain of memory loss and difficulty with concentration.

Severe anxiety or hypochondriacal states are rare over 65 years.

Management

BIOLOGICAL

Once the clinical diagnosis has been made, it is essential to exclude potentially reversible causes of dementia. Basic investigations include full blood count, erythrocyte sedimentation rate (ESR), urea and electrolytes, liver function tests, thyroid function tests, B_{12} and folate, chest X-ray, and ECG. CT scan or MRI is helpful to exclude space-occupying lesion and subdural haematoma. Also consider physical treatments such as low-dose sedating neuroleptics (e.g. thioridazine) for insomnia, restlessness, agitation, paranoia and/or aggressive behaviour. If markedly depressed consider an antidepressant, e.g. lofepramine. Beware overuse of drugs: remember cardiovascular side-effects and possibility of falls.

SOCIAL
The main aim of effective care is to provide good, safe physical care in an environment that is familiar to the individual for as long as possible. It is important to provide support for family and carers as well as the individual with dementia. Respite care may be greatly welcomed.

PSYCHOLOGICAL
The aim is to allow the individual with dementia to maintain their self-esteem, thus avoiding traumatic catastrophic reactions. Such measures include discussions of past and current events, visible means of orientation and highly structured daily activities.

DELIRIUM (ICD-10 F05)

Definition

Acute organic brain dysfunction, characterized by disturbance of consciousness and attention, perception, thinking, memory, psychomotor activity and emotion that is transient and of fluctuating intensity. Unlike dementia (see p. 192) delirium is almost always non-progressive and reversible.

Clinical features

- Impairment of consciousness and attention. Disorientation for time, place and sometimes for person. Inability to attend to one stimulus for a prolonged period

- Illusions, hallucinations, and delusional beliefs. Usually transient, fragmented and poorly systematized. Hallucinations may be visual as well as auditory

- Restlessness, overactivity and agitation. May however show signs of hypo-activity and psychomotor retardation. Speech may be increased or decreased

- Impairment of registration: very poor short-term memory

- Emotional disturbance: depression, anxiety, and fearfulness are common. Mood may appear quite labile. Perplexity and suspiciousness are also seen

- Disturbance of sleep–wake cycle: manifests as insomnia, reversal of diurnal cycle, daytime drowsiness and worsening of symptoms at night

- Other signs of cerebral dysfunction including dysphasia, apraxia, and dysgraphia

The onset of delirium is usually rapid.

Epidemiology

Seen most often in the elderly (>60 years) and among hospital patients. Reported to occur in 10% of medical patients, 20% of burns patients and 30% of ITU patients. 'Chronic' delirium lasting for 6 months or more has been observed among patients with chronic liver disease, carcinoma and subacute bacterial endocarditis. A previous episode of delirium significantly increases the risk of future delirium.

Basic science

Delirium is almost always due to an underlying systemic organic disturbance. Common causes include:

- Infections: e.g. respiratory or urinary tract infections, cellulitis and septicaemia
- Cardiovascular disturbance: arrhythmias, blood loss or anaemia (e.g. post-operative)
- Respiratory distress or hypoxia
- Metabolic disturbances: hypoglycaemia, renal or liver failure, severe vitamin deficiency
- Neoplasms

Differential diagnosis

- Dementia (see p. 192)
- Acute psychotic disorders including schizophrenia and mania

- Acute intoxication: drugs, alcohol or poisons including Wernicke's encephalopathy (see p. 224)
- Acute withdrawal from drugs or alcohol
- Temporal lobe epilepsy and post-ictal states
- Dissociative states

Management

The most important aspect of management is the identification of the cause of delirium. Many of the causes of delirium are life-threatening medical emergencies. Since the delirious patient is behaviourally disturbed it is easy to misdiagnose a primary psychiatric disorder. It is therefore imperative to physically examine and investigate any patient who is disorientated for time and place.

PHYSICAL EXAMINATION should look for evidence of focal sepsis, trauma, cardiac, renal or hepatic failure. Investigations should include urgent full blood count, urea and electrolytes, glucose, ESR, chest X-ray and blood cultures if pyrexial. EEG and CT scan are indicated if neurological signs are elicited or if no cause is found and symptoms persist.

MEDICAL CARE should concentrate on treating the underlying cause of the delirium. Small amounts of neuroleptic medication (e.g. chlorpromazine) may help behavioural disturbances including agitation and restlessness, as well as emotional lability, hallucinations and frightening illusions.

SKILLED NURSING CARE is imperative. The delirious patient requires one-to-one nursing in a quiet but well-lit room. Staff should expect that the symptoms of delirium are likely to be worse at night than during the day.

SCHIZOPHRENIA

Definition

The most common psychotic disorder, schizophrenia is characterized by abnormalities in perception, beliefs, thought processing and expression, volition, and reality testing. The phenomenology of schizophrenia can be divided into acute and chronic features.

Clinical features

Acute illness

Auditory hallucinations: though both second- and third-person auditory hallucinations occur, it is the latter which are of diagnostic importance. Third-person auditory hallucinations are characteristically described as two or more people discussing the patient, often in a derogatory manner; also experience third-person commentary in which the patient hears someone describing their actions as they are carried out, and *echo de la pensée* in which the patient can hear their own thoughts aloud.

Somatic (bodily) hallucinations: though diagnostically significant, these are less common than auditory hallucinations.

Delusional beliefs are very common, particularly those with persecutory content. The most important diagnostically, and also the rarest, are primary delusions, in which a fully formed belief suddenly occurs 'out of the blue'. Ideas of reference are also very common in schizophrenia, in which unrelated notices, signs or remarks are believed to be messages with specific meaning for the patient. Ideas of reference are often found in the media, and usually involve a tangential connection with the subject.

Thought insertion/withdrawal/broadcast, in which the patient believes that others know what they are thinking, either because these can be heard aloud (akin to *echo de la pensée*) or are transmitted through radio or television. Most likely to represent both delusional beliefs and auditory hallucinations.

Passivity experiences in which the patient feels that their bodily functions, emotions or thoughts are under external control. The most important diagnostically is thought block, in which a train of thought comes to a sudden halt, accompanied by the experience of having the thought removed from the patient's mind.

Formal thought disorder whereby an individual has difficulty expressing their own thoughts. In mild thought disorder an individual has trouble maintaining a train of thought (loosening of association), and may appear to 'go off at a tangent', or talk past the point (*vorbereiden*). When more severe this results in disjunctures in thought, or 'knight's move' thinking (or derailment). When very severe words become jumbled up in a 'word salad' (verbigeration), which may contain examples of words invented by the individual (neologisms).

Individuals with acute schizophrenia may be highly suspicious, aroused and irritable, or grandiose.

Chronic symptoms

Also referred to as 'negative symptoms', the symptoms of chronic schizophrenia include affective blunting, apathy, poverty of thought and speech, social withdrawal, and self-neglect. Although the acute symptoms are extremely distressing, and may lead to potentially life-threatening behaviour, it is the chronic symptoms that are responsible for impairment and handicap.

Epidemiology

Lifetime risk is about 1% in the general population. In the UK prevalence is about 0.5–1% and incidence about 14 per 100 000 per year. There is no sex difference in prevalence. The first onset typically is between 15 and 45 years, although men exhibit symptoms earlier than women.

Prevalence is highest in low socioeconomic status groups, among the unmarried and in urban areas. Although these findings have traditionally been explained in terms of 'social drift', this has been challenged by recent findings.

In the UK, rates in first-generation immigrants from the Caribbean are higher than in the indigenous population (about 2:1), but are higher still in second-generation African Caribbeans (about 10:1). The latter finding has yet to be explained.

Findings which support a neurodevelopmental model of schizophrenia are associations between schizophrenia and season of birth, obstetric complications, and maternal exposure to either influenza epidemics or starvation during the first and/or second trimesters of pregnancy.

Despite similar rates of incidence around the world, the outcome of schizophrenia appears to be significantly better in developing countries than in North America or Europe.

Basic science

Recent developments in neuroimaging have established that there are structural and functional brain abnormalities in schizophrenia, though none are considered to be pathognomonic. Chief among the structural changes are lateral ventricular enlargement, a diminution in the size of the frontal lobes, particularly the amygdala, hippocampus and parahippocampal gyrus. Thickening of the corpus callosum has also been reported.

Important functional changes, detected by studies of local blood flow and neuronal activity, have demonstrated not only that there is reduced activity in the frontal lobes ('hypofrontality') but also that auditory hallucinations are associated with increased activity in Broca's area, a part of the brain normally associated with speech production. The advent of MRI, and more recently functional MRI, has led to a renewed interest in the neuroanatomy and neurophysiology of schizophrenia.

The dominant neuropharmacological model of schizophrenia is still based on the dopamine hypothesis, in which the symptoms of this disorder are accounted for by a relative excess of dopamine.

Twin and family studies indicate that there is a strong genetic component in the aetiology of schizophrenia. Concordance rates in monozygotic (MZ) twins are about 50%, compared with 10% in dizygotic (DZ) twins. The lifetime risk of schizophrenia is increased by about 10 times in siblings of probands, 12 times in children of one schizophrenic parent and 50 times in children of two schizophrenic parents. Adoption studies have found that children of schizophrenics have significantly higher rates of schizophrenia than members of the family into which they are adopted. Results from molecular genetic studies indicate that the predisposition to schizophrenia is likely to involve several genes, rather than just one.

It has been suggested that there are two aetiological 'types' of schizophrenia, one which is inherited ('genetic'), and one which occurs because of a 'brain injury' suffered at a developmentally sensitive stage. Despite sound evidence of pre-morbid developmental abnormalities during childhood and adolescence, the 'neurodevelopmental' model of schizophrenia has yet to be substantiated.

Differential diagnosis

Psychiatric

- Mania. Though the symptoms often overlap, mania is characterized by prominent affective component (elation, grandiosity, disinhibition, overactivity, irritability and lability of mood), while acute schizophrenia is characterized most often by suspicion, paranoia or perplexity.

- Depression. Chronic schizophrenia may mimic or coexist with depression, particularly in young people and those who retain insight into the nature of their illness.

Organic

Includes very rare conditions such as Huntington's chorea, Wilson's disease, temporal lobe epilepsy, frontal or temporal lobe tumour, early multiple sclerosis, early systemic lupus erythematosus (SLE), porphyria, and substance abuse (especially LSD, ecstasy, amphetamines and cocaine/crack).

Management

Studies in the UK, Australia and the USA have shown that patients with both acute and chronic schizophrenia can be cared for satisfactorily outside traditional psychiatric hospital inpatient settings. However, while this community-based care has proved significantly less costly than inpatient treatment, and is preferred by patients and their carers, there is no evidence of any clinical or social outcome differences.

Management of acute schizophrenia

The first priority is to ensure the safety of the patient and others. Despite media coverage to the contrary, schizophrenic patients are more likely to be the victims of violent crime than its perpetrators. Though rarely homicidal, patients with schizophrenia are at high risk of suicide, and careful assessment of risk is mandatory. This should involve discussion with informants.

The mainstay of treatment is pharmacological, in the form of neuroleptic medication. These may be administered orally, intramuscularly or in an emergency (to achieve rapid tranquillization), intravenously. The most sedating neuroleptic is chlorpromazine. Some patients may benefit from augmentation of neuroleptics with diazepam (for a short time) if aroused, lithium carbonate if associated with prominent affective symptoms, or carbamazepine if aggressive.

While most acute (positive) symptoms can be controlled with regular doses of the older neuroleptic drugs, some are resistant to such treatment, even at high doses. A proportion of these individuals will respond to newer antipsychotics, including risperidone and clozapine. The latter may sometimes produce dramatic results, but requires careful monitoring because of the risk of agranulocytosis.

Management of chronic schizophrenia

Rehabilitation aims to allow the patient to lead as near normal a life as possible, and incorporates relapse prevention. Effective rehabilitation addresses all aspects of social, psychological, and emotional functioning.

Relapse prevention may be achieved by (i) ensuring compliance with medication, (ii) assertive aftercare coordinated by a keyworker, and (iii) support and education for relatives and other carers.

Since patients with schizophrenia often lack insight into their condition, many cease compliance with medication at the earliest opportunity. The use of depot injections is a partial solution, since it allows medication to be given only every 3–4 weeks. A recent development is the use of so-called motivational interviews to enhance insight and therefore compliance with medication.

Domiciliary visiting of patients who default from treatment, or who fail to attend clinic appointments may increase the chance of compliance with medication, but certainly facilitates early intervention when signs of relapse do occur.

There is very strong evidence that supportive psychoeducational family therapy can significantly reduce the rate of relapse, particularly in patients who are also compliant with prophylactic medication. The main aim of this type of treatment is to help families to understand more about this illness, and to minimize the chance of over-stimulation at home. Research indicates that criticism, over-involvement and prolonged face-to-face contact with other family members are all associated with high rates of both arousal and subsequent recurrence of psychotic symptoms.

Rehabilitation requires a formal assessment of both individual skills in activities of daily living (ADL) (cooking, cleaning, washing, personal hygiene and budgeting), usually by an occupational therapist, housing and financial circumstances, and the availability, ability and attitudes of informal carers. Patients may need help with some or all of these; if severely disabled they may need to live in supported accommodation.

Previous models of rehabilitation incorporated graded hierarchies of residential and occupational settings, through which individual patients would move when they were able. Day centres offering mixtures of structured occupational therapy and informal opportunities to socialize have largely replaced sheltered workshops. Most areas have a range of different types of supported accommodation, though most are owned and operated by voluntary organizations, such as housing associations, and are funded by social services and housing benefit payments. Supported accommodation ranges from nursing homes staffed 24 hours a day by qualified nurses, through hostels staffed by care assistants in which there may be a member of staff on site at night, to supported group homes or flats in which residents are visited by non-resident staff.

AFFECTIVE DISORDERS

Definition

Two types of mood disorder are recognized by categorical systems of classification – mania and depression – though in reality these probably exist as extremes on a continuum. Both ICD-10 and DSM-IV abound with different ways of classifying depression. For the present purposes we distinguish only between the psychotic disorders (manic-depressive psychosis and psychotic depression) and unipolar, non-psychotic depression. Though manic-depressive psychosis may first present with a manic episode, one or more episodes of depression invariably follow. 'Unipolar' mania is extremely uncommon.

Clinical features of mania (ICD-10 F30.0)

Although described as a persistent excessive elevation of mood, patients suffering from mania commonly present in a so-called mixed affective state, with lability of mood and features of both 'classical' mania and depression. Manic episodes generally develop over 1 or 2 days, culminating in disinhibition, overactivity and increasingly uncontrollable behaviour. Patients with acute mania may do themselves great harm through overspending and sexual disinhibition, and are prone to physical exhaustion. Mania is by definition a psychotic condition.

- Elevation of mood, characterized by overactivity, euphoria, grandiosity, and increased libido

- Thought disorder including pressure of speech, flight of ideas, puns, and clang associations (rhyming)

- Restlessness, insomnia and irritability, intolerance of frustration and persistent demands. May lead to aggression and/or violence
- Lack of insight and diminished judgement, which combined with the above symptoms may lead to, for example, overspending or unprotected sexual intercourse, occurrences that may have consequences extending beyond the duration of the acute manic episode
- Hallucinations, most commonly auditory but also in other sensory modalities
- Delusional beliefs and ideas of reference, particularly involving grandiose and/or persecutory themes

Note that Schneider's first-rank symptoms of schizophrenia occur in about 20% of patients with mania.

Clinical features of depression (ICD-10 F32)

In contrast to mania, depression is only rarely associated with psychotic symptoms. The signs and symptoms of depression are often considered under the following headings.

Physical (or 'vegetative')

- Poor sleep (insomnia): this may take the form of initial insomnia, broken sleep and/or early morning waking. The latter is the most significant diagnostically. Occasionally depressed subjects (especially those with 'atypical' depression and/or seasonal affective disorder, SAD) report hypersomnia. Even when they do sleep, depressed patients characteristically complain of not feeling rested or refreshed on waking

- Fatigue/anergia
- Poor appetite and weight loss. Like sleep, some depressed patients (e.g. SAD) report increased appetite (especially for carbohydrate-rich food) and weight gain
- Diurnal variation of mood: depressed patients typically report feeling worse first thing in the morning
- Psychomotor retardation *or* agitation: the latter is a very dangerous sign, since agitated patients are at high risk of self-harm, which they may attempt out of desperation
- Dehydration and/or constipation especially in the elderly
- Loss of libido

Psychological

- Low mood
- Anhedonia (inability to experience pleasure)
- Self-blame and guilt
- Feelings of hopelessness and pessimism about the future
- Irritability
- Suicidal ideation

Cognitive

- Poor concentration and increased distractibility

- Memory impairment
- Memory appears selective for 'unhappy' events
- Negative self-appraisal/self-criticism

Depression may be accompanied by psychotic symptoms, the nature and content of which are almost always mood congruent. These most commonly take the form of auditory hallucinations, often in the second person, and delusions, which typically have a negative or nihilistic content (e.g. that the patient's insides are rotting).

For a diagnosis of severe depression (F32.2), all three of the 'core' depressive symptoms must be present, namely depressed mood, loss of interest and enjoyment (anhedonia) and increased fatiguability, plus at least four other symptoms. A severe depressive episode should be of at least 2 weeks' duration.

Epidemiology

Manic-depressive psychosis

Lifetime risk of manic-depressive psychosis is about 0.5–1% in the general population. Prevalence of acute mania is about 0.5%. No clear sex or socioeconomic differences in prevalence or incidence of mania or manic-depressive psychosis. First onset of mania/manic-depressive psychosis usually occurs before 30 years, earlier than the onset of unipolar (non-psychotic) depression.

Unipolar depression

Prevalence of major depression is about 2–3% of the general population. Prevalence of moderate and mild depression is about 10–15%. Though less severe, mild depression accounts for about twice as many days of lost employment as major depression, owing to the higher prevalence.

Incidence of major depression is about 1–2% per year in the general population. Incidence of moderate and mild depression is about 5–10% per year.

The highest prevalence is in women (female:male about 2:1). Recent evidence indicates that this is due to a higher incidence of depression among women, rather than longer duration of individual episodes. Most evidence indicates that this sex difference is likely to be social in origin, rather than the result of genetic differences, or differences in sex hormones. There is some evidence that the sex difference in prevalence is greatest between the ages of 20 and 60 years, when men's and women's social roles are most clearly differentiated.

Prevalence is highest among those with the lowest socioeconomic status, although findings concerning occupational social class have been inconsistent. There is clear evidence that these disorders are strongly associated with measures of low material standard of living, including low income, living in rented accommodation and not having access to a car. Recent studies indicate that these associations are unlikely to be explained by social selection (i.e. downward social mobility).

Higher rates are also found in the unemployed, those with little or no education, and those who are separated, divorced or widowed.

Basic science

Manic-depressive psychosis runs in families, and there is evidence that this is due to a genetic effect. MZ/DZ concordance rates are about 4:1 (80% vs. 20%). The heritability of manic-depressive psychosis has been estimated to be 86%. Although there is no consistent evidence concerning specific genetic mechanisms, recent suggestions have included genes on chromosome 11 (reported in a large Amish family), and X-linked dominance with incomplete penetrance.

A genetic contribution has also been identified for unipolar major depression. A recent epidemiological twin study in the USA estimated that genetic factors accounted for 11% of the variance in liability to major depression, compared with recent life events (15%), past history of major depression (9%), neuroticism (6%), 'recent difficulties' (including financial hardship) (4%), and lack of parental warmth (4%).

While it has been shown consistently that threatening life events in the preceding 3 months are causally associated with the incidence of depression, there is also evidence that this association may be modified by material circumstances, occupational social class, self-esteem, childhood experiences and social support, particularly that elicited at times of crisis.

Theories concerning the mechanisms within the brain by which the symptoms of mania and depression arise have concentrated on noradrenaline (NA) and serotonin (5-HT). According to the simplest version of the amine hypothesis, depressive symptoms are associated with low levels of NA and 5-HT, and manic symptoms with an excess of these transmitters. While this hypothesis is partially supported by the finding of low levels of 3-methoxy-4-hydroxyphenylglycol (MHPG; metabolite of NA) in the urine of depressed subjects, low levels of 5-HT and 5-HT metabolites in suicides (post-mortem), there are also inconsistencies, including the unexplained delay in the onset of clinical response to anti-depressants.

215

VIII: SPECIFIC CONDITIONS

Differential diagnosis of mania

Organic

- Frontal lobe syndromes, associated with disinhibition, thought disorder, inappropriate affective responses and chaotic behaviour. Possible causes include tumours, infection, trauma and degenerative diseases such as Pick's disease
- Drug-induced mania, such as may be precipitated by steroids, amphetamines, cocaine and hallucinogens
- Multiple sclerosis
- Temporal lobe epilepsy
- Wilson's disease
- Hyperthyroidism

Psychiatric

Schizophrenia may be difficult to exclude in the presence of Schneiderian first-rank symptoms. Important diagnostic features include family psychiatric history (i.e. tendency for different conditions to 'breed true'), past psychiatric history (though schizophrenia can also be associated with features of depression) and degree of symptomatic recovery between episodes. Note past controversy over concepts such as 'unitary psychosis' and 'schizo-affective disorders'.

Differential diagnosis of depression

Organic

- Endocrine disorders: Cushing's disease, hypothyroidism, hyperparathyroidism
- Drugs including alcohol, corticosteroids, methyldopa, propranolol, cimetidine and amphetamine withdrawal
- Head injury
- Neoplasms particularly carcinoma of pancreas, brain and lung
- Malnutrition, regardless of cause (including anorexia). May be mediated by B_{12} deficiency
- Dementia, which may mimic depression (and vice versa)
- Post-viral fatigue, though the status of this diagnosis remains in doubt

Note that with the exception of dementia, all of the above represent organic *causes* of depression.

Psychiatric

- Schizophrenia
- Alcohol dependency syndrome
- Obsessive–compulsive disorder
- Generalized anxiety disorder

Note that all of these may either mimic depression, or coexist with depression as either a primary or secondary psychiatric condition. Indeed, it is extremely rare for depression to occur in the absence of significant anxiety.

Management of affective disorders

Management of mania

ACUTE MANAGEMENT

Assess carefully and tactfully. Manic patients are often poor historians, and are usually impatient, terminating interviews without warning. Always try to get an account of recent events from an informant. Beware irritability and quick temper – make sure backup is available. Most important information: any recent drug use, any current physical health problems, plus past psychiatric history and treatment. Does patient normally take lithium? Important to ask about psychotic symptoms, plus understanding of current illness (insight) and willingness to accept treatment.

If not psychotic, willing to accept treatment, no danger to him/herself or others, and supported in the community, consider treating as an out-patient. In the short term best treatment is neuroleptic medication, e.g. chlorpromazine 100–200 mg daily. Patients who have stopped taking lithium recently should be strongly recommended to recommence this medication. The main limitation of this approach is that manic patients characteristically lack insight, and compliance with medication is often inconsistent.

If psychotic, uncompliant, unsupported or judged to be dangerous (including risk of further deterioration in the patient's own health), admission is mandatory. Medication should be commenced at once. Neuroleptic medication may be augmented by benzodiazepines and/or lithium. Such patients will require intensive nursing care, and may also need rapid tranquillization (see p. 27) during the acute phase of their illness, especially as they may be very aroused by being forcibly detained in hospital.

Patients unresponsive to the above may benefit from ECT.

RELAPSE PREVENTION

The mainstay of relapse prevention is the prescription of mood-stabilizing drugs, namely lithium, carbamezepine and (less commonly) sodium valproate. Other drugs which are believed to act in this way are clonazepam and verapamil.

Patients with this disorder need counselling about the likely prognosis, the importance of maintaining compliance with their medication, and 'early warning signs' indicative of relapse (such as initial insomnia). If such features can be identified it may be possible to formulate an 'emergency' strategy to be implemented in the case of relapse, since some patients retain insight in the prodromal stages of an acute episode of mania. Besides this supportive psychotherapy, recovered patients may also require considerable practical assistance in returning to the community, where they must repair any financial, physical and emotional damage done in the acute phase of their illness.

Although some centres attempt psychodynamic psychotherapy with patients with a history of manic-depressive psychosis, this type of intervention may precipitate manic relapses and is generally viewed as a contraindication for this type of treatment.

Management of depression

ACUTE MANAGEMENT

If psychotic and/or suicidal, patient requires admission. The first priority in management is the patient's safety, and continuous nursing observation is mandatory. Important to ask about current suicidal thoughts and plans, and previous attempts at suicidal or deliberate self-harm, and any family history of suicide. Agitated patients are at high risk of self-harm.

The first line of treatment in severe depression is a tricyclic antidepressant, unless contraindicated. The main contraindications are coexisting cardiac disease including recent myocardial infarction or arrhythmias and intolerance of anticholinergic side-effects (e.g. urinary retention). Among tricyclic drugs, the choice is between those which are more or less sedating. Thus, amitriptyline and dothiepin are much more sedating than imipramine, desipramine and lofepramine. In addition, lofepramine has a weaker anticholinergic effect and is far safer in overdose than other tricyclics. (Note that it is not yet known at what level of severity of depression the benefits of such treatment outweigh the drawbacks.)

The main alternatives to tricyclic drugs are the SSRIs such as fluoxetine and sertraline, which do not have anticholinergic side-effects, are not sedating, and are safe in overdose. There is no evidence that SSRIs are any more effective than tricyclics. The main side-effects of these drugs are nausea, diarrhoea and agitation. One advantage of starting with a tricyclic drug is that a drug-free interval of 1 week is required when changing from an SSRI to a tricyclic.

Neither class of antidepressant has an antidepressant effect for the first 10–14 days.

If the patient does not respond to 6 weeks of treatment on a therapeutic dose of a tricyclic (equivalent to 150 mg amitriptyline for 4 weeks) or an SSRI (e.g. fluoxetine 20 mg for 4 weeks), consider increasing the dose of current medication or changing to an antidepressant of a different class. If this fails, augmentation with lithium or L-thyronine may help. Little is known about the effects of combination treatment with a tricyclic and an SSRI.

Neuroleptic medication, such as thioridazine, should be used if the depression is accompanied by psychotic symptoms. This drug is also very effective in treating any agitation, particularly among the elderly where this is a not infrequent feature.

ECT is indicated in the management of resistant depression and where antidepressants are contraindicated (e.g. some elderly patients), or when the patient's life may be at risk (from suicide or dehydration, arising from a refusal to eat or drink).

Psychological treatments: cognitive therapy (see p. 324) appears to be as effective as antidepressant medication in treating the acute phase of moderate and severe depression.

RELAPSE PREVENTION

Depression is a relapsing and remitting disorder, and those who have suffered even a single episode are at greatly increased risk of future episodes.

It is recommended that any antidepressant medication should be continued for a minimum of 6 months after the resolution of the acute episode.

Cognitive therapy appears to be superior to antidepressant treatment in preventing relapse. Some individuals who have suffered from depression may be suitable for individual or group psychodynamic psychotherapy. This type of treatment requires a significant investment of time (and sometimes money) on the part of the patient, and definitive evidence of clinical effectiveness has yet to be demonstrated.

SUBSTANCE MISUSE

Definition

The definition of drug dependence includes the occurrence of withdrawal symptoms, drug use for the relief of withdrawal symptoms, subjective awareness of an inability to control drug-taking behaviour, increasing tolerance to the psychoactive properties of the drug over time, narrowing of the repertoire of drug consumption, salience of drug-taking over other activities, persistent drug use despite evidence of harm, and rapid reinstatement of drug taking after periods of abstinence.

Alcohol and other drug dependencies share many common features in terms of aetiology, prognosis and management, and are therefore considered together. Other commonly misused substances are cannabis, opiates, stimulants, hypnotics and tranquillizers, hallucinogens and solvents.

We discuss here only dependence with alcohol, opiates and stimulants. Though the specific physical and psychiatric complications may vary, the general principles underlying the management of dependency is the same for most drugs.

Clinical features of alcohol dependency

Psychiatric complications

Delirium tremens occurs about 72 hours after withdrawal. Characterized by tremor, restlessness, disorientation, visual hallucinations (though auditory or somatic hallucinations may also occur), autonomic arousal (fever, tachycardia, sweating) and occasionally fits. Though self-limiting over 72–96 hours, it should not be left untreated since mortality is about 10%. For this reason alcohol-dependent patients should be advised not to withdraw from alcohol without medical supervision.

Depression is common, and may reflect the pharmacological action of alcohol, a common genetic predisposition to both depression and alcohol dependency, or a psychological response to awareness of the addiction and the damage this has inflicted on the physical, psychological and social well-being of the patient and their family. The risk of suicide is 50 times higher in those who are dependent on alcohol than in the rest of the population.

Alcoholic hallucinosis describes (usually) auditory hallucinations in the context of clear consciousness. These are not associated with withdrawal, and usually begin while subjects are still drinking. Hallucinations often cease if abstinence is maintained for 6 months or longer. Neuroleptic medication is indicated if these persist despite abstinence from alcohol.

Suspiciousness, irritability and pathological jealousy. The patient may develop a delusional belief that their partner or spouse has been unfaithful. Escalates from suspicion to interrogation, surveillance and, not infrequently, violence. Very dangerous.

Cognitive impairment affects more than 50% of alcohol-dependent patients seen by psychiatrists, manifesting as deficits in short-term memory and learning, as well as a reduced capacity for adapting to novel circumstances, suggestive of frontal lobe damage. This brain damage reduces the capacity for initiating and maintaining abstinence from alcohol. A related phenomenon is episodic amnesia for events during periods of drunkenness.

Korsakoff's syndrome is a rare but severe, largely irreversible impairment of short-term memory associated with confabulation, due to necrosis in the mammillary bodies. May appear on resolution of Wernicke's encephalopathy.

Physical complications

- Increased mortality. Men who report consuming 6 or more units per day experience mortality three times greater than men who consume less than this amount, a difference which is partly accounted for by heavier smoking, suicide and accidental deaths

- Liver damage (alcoholic liver disease), leading to hepatitis, cirrhosis and cancer of the liver

- Gastrointestinal complaints including gastritis, peptic ulceration, haematemesis and diarrhoea, plus cancer of the oropharynx, oesophagus and stomach

- Malnutrition, including thiamine deficiency

- Pneumonia and/or tuberculosis associated with poverty and/or homelessness

- Pancreatitis, progressing to fibrosis and calcification (chronic relapsing pancreatitis)

- Diabetes mellitus

- Cushing's syndrome

- Cardiovascular disease including athero-sclerosis, hypertension, arrhythmias and cardiomyopathy, though 1–3 units of alcohol per day appear to reduce the risk of coronary artery disease
- Sexual impairment resulting from organic impotence, reduced libido, anxiety and dysfunctional relationships
- Wernicke's encephalopathy is characterized by confusion, ataxia and ocular palsy, arising from haemorrhages in the brainstem and hypothalamus. High mortality, and survivors likely to develop Korsakoff's syndrome (see above). Differential diagnosis is subdural haematoma
- 'Blackouts', i.e. loss of consciousness when intoxicated
- Polyneuropathy due to vitamin deficiencies, leading to flaccid weakness which starts in lower limbs with a characteristic stocking distribution
- Fetal alcohol syndrome

Social damage

At worst, dependency becomes a downward spiral culminating in 'park bench' destitution. Steps along the way may include unemployment, breakdown of marital and other family relationships, poverty, homelessness and crime, including drunk driving offences.

Clinical features of opiate dependency

Opiates (e.g. morphine, heroin, pethidine, methadone, dihydrocodeine, buprenorphine) create a detached, pain-free, dream-like state and induce physical dependency very rapidly. The main psychiatric complications associated with opiate use are due to (1) the salience of drug-seeking behaviour, (2) needle sharing, and (3) the difficulty and expense of obtaining a regular supply.

Physical complications

Injecting is a major source of physical morbidity. In addition to this, the composition of 'street' drugs varies greatly.

- Increased mortality: heroin addicts are 16 times more likely to die than other people of the same age. One major cause of premature death is overdose

- Overdose presents as pupillary constriction, respiratory depression, bradycardia, nausea and vomiting, slurred speech and hypothermia. *This is a medical emergency*

- Hepatitis, HIV infection and AIDS among injecters

- Withdrawal symptoms, though subjectively unpleasant, are much less life-threatening than withdrawal from alcohol. Symptoms increase in intensity over 48 hours and include abdominal cramps, diarrhoea, nausea and vomiting, rhinorrhoea, lacrimation, sweating and yawning. Note that piloerection is a sign that cannot be mimicked

- Malnutrition

- Pneumonia and/or tuberculosis associated with poverty and/or homelessness

- Thrombophlebitis and/or skin abscesses due to injecting

- Infectious endocarditis (subacute bacterial endocarditis) due to injecting

Social damage

- Unemployment
- Homelessness
- Crime: unlike alcohol, which is legal but may be associated with criminal behaviour, opiate addicts almost always need to engage in criminal activities simply to fund their habit. Though some addicts achieve this by supplying drugs to others (in a sort of pyramid), the most common crimes are probably shoplifting and house breaking. Among women prostitution is a major problem, since this carries significant health risks.

Clinical features of stimulant dependency

These drugs include amphetamine, dextroamphetamine, methamphetamine, cocaine and 'crack' cocaine.

Psychiatric complications

Acute intoxication with stimulants is characterized by restlessness, alertness, agitation, pressure of speech and insomnia. May be difficult to distinguish from mania. Though euphoria is common, some individuals become suspicious, aggressive, irritable and even violent. The latter is found most commonly among those who use crack cocaine. These symptoms are accompanied by signs of autonomic arousal, including tachycardia, hypertension, tremulousness and pupillary dilation. Crack cocaine has a very rapid onset of action ('rush'), which is of relatively brief duration. The characteristic rebound dysphoria leads to repeated use and dependency.

Acute confusional state (delirium), shortly after consuming drug. May be accompanied by violence.

Acute paranoid psychosis ('amphetamine psychosis') occurs in the context of clear consciousness. Accompanied by anxiety, hostility, suspiciousness, agitation and ideas of reference. Resembles paranoid schizophrenia. Variable time course.

Depression may occur with prolonged use, or on withdrawal from amphetamines. The latter is accompanied by fatigue, anxiety and insomnia.

Physical complications

- Convulsions in those taking large doses, may result in (possibly fatal) anoxia
- Myocardial ischaemia, leading to myocardial infarction
- Cerebrovascular accidents
- Malnutrition and pneumonia
- Ischaemia and necrosis of the nasal septum arising from repeated inhalation of cocaine, a drug which is also a potent vasoconstrictor

Social damage

These are similar to those described for alcohol and opiates, and include crime (including prostitution), poverty, homelessness, and breakdown of close relationships.

Management of substance misuse

Medical and psychiatric emergencies

DELIRIUM TREMENS

Management involves admission to hospital and nursing care in well-lit uncluttered surroundings. Appropriate investigations are full blood count, urea and electrolytes and liver function tests. Treatment includes parenteral vitamin B_6 (thiamine) first, followed by correction of dehydration. If fits cannot be controlled with benzodiazepines (e.g. diazepam) orally or parenterally, try an intravenous infusion of chlormethiazole. If no fits occur, or after fits have been controlled, a reducing dose of a benzodiazepine, e.g. chlordiazepoxide, is recommended for the first 7–10 days of abstinence.

If level of consciousness fluctuates, consider possibility of subdural haematoma or Wernicke's encephalopathy (see above). Treatment of the latter includes intravenous thiamine and supportive care.

OPIATE OVERDOSE

Characterized by loss of consciousness, shallow breathing and pupillary constriction (though pupils may be dilated if cerebral anoxia has occurred). High mortality due to respiratory depression and pulmonary oedema. Needs intensive medical treatment. First-line management is i.v. naloxone, an opiate antagonist, given up to five times over 15 minutes. If no response, coma probably not due to opiate overdose. If positive response continue to monitor as patient may need further doses of naloxone. Remember that naloxone will produce symptoms of opiate withdrawal in dependent individuals.

ACUTE PARANOID PSYCHOSIS (especially associated with stimulant use)

Diagnosis may be made clinically, especially if there is a history of drug use. Although most stimulants can be detected in urine, it is often very difficult to obtain a sample. Acute management involves standard treatment of agitation, delirium or psychosis, including reassurance and careful nursing. Short-term use of a benzodiazepine may be useful if agitated or anxious, while psychotic symptoms should be treated with a neuroleptic such as haloperidol. Particular attention must be given to issues of safety, since intoxicated and withdrawing patients may be violent and/or suicidal. Remember also that stimulant use increases risk of cerebrovascular accident and myocardial infarction.

Managing withdrawal

ALCOHOL
As has been pointed out, unmedicated withdrawal from alcohol is not recommended for those who are dependent in view of the risk of convulsions. Withdrawal from alcohol can be safely achieved under medical supervision over 7–10 days, on an outpatient basis. A reducing dose of a benzodiazepine, e.g. chlordiazepoxide, should be used to control withdrawal symptoms during this period. Though this drug is relatively safe if taken with alcohol, it is usually recommended that patients collect their medication on a daily basis, when they may also be breathalysed to confirm abstinence. Since many people who are dependent on alcohol are also depressed, it should also be possible to ascertain whether an antidepressant is indicated.

OPIATES

Note that all new cases of opiate abuse must be notified to the Home Office. Withdrawal is managed using reducing doses of methadone titrated against severity of withdrawal symptoms. Unlike alcohol withdrawal, opiate withdrawal is rarely life-threatening. Most withdrawals take 7–10 days. Maintenance prescriptions of methadone are sometimes provided for patients who are unable to withdraw from opiates, though this remains a minority practice. Pragmatic risk minimization strategies, such as needle-exchange programmes, have been widely adopted by drug-treatment centres given the major health and social risks associated with continued drug use.

MAINTAINING ABSTINENCE

This is the key to reducing the prevalence of substance abuse, and also the most difficult to achieve. All types of substance abuse occur within a social context, and there is good evidence that the likelihood of lapse and relapse are extremely high if this remains unchanged. However effective the management of withdrawal, substance use is frequently reinstated in response to familiar cues, such as familiar off-licences, pubs and peers. Days may be very difficult to fill for the newly abstinent, in the absence of drugs or alcohol, and the routine associated with their acquisition and consumption. Thus, though difficult, the best way to maintain abstinence is to convince the patient to alter his or her social context. For some individuals, this may involve help with rehousing and employment training. Abstinence may also be reinforced through peer support and self-scrutiny (e.g. Alcoholics Anonymous), group psychotherapy, family therapy, support for relatives and social skills training. A very important message is that 'controlled' substance use (e.g. just having one drink) almost inevitably leads to a reinstatement of dependency.

NEUROTIC DISORDERS
(ICD-10 F40-48)

Although psychiatrists traditionally subdivide the non-psychotic disorders into a series of distinct clinical entities, pure examples of these disorders are rare in community settings. Epidemiological evidence indicates that anxiety and depression are highly correlated, and the majority of 'cases' have a combination of both types of symptom (i.e. mixed anxiety/depression). The more severe disorders are found most commonly in psychiatric settings, where it is possible to distinguish between (primary) depression, generalized anxiety disorder, phobias and panic disorder, and obsessive–compulsive disorder. With the exception of 'pure' depression (and the extent to which this occurs is debatable), all of the neurotic disorders are characterized by the experience of anxiety, to a greater or lesser degree.

Clinical features

Anxiety

- Ideational: fear and apprehension
- Somatic symptoms of autonomic arousal, including sweating, dry mouth, palpita-

tions, hyperventilation, tremor, headache, backache, flushing, nausea, diarrhoea, urinary frequency. These symptoms may mimic cardiovascular disease, particularly if accompanied by chest pain. Also sensation of muscular tension. These symptoms may be exacerbated by hyperventilation/overbreathing, which may also result in dizziness, peri-oral and limb paraesthesiae, and muscular spasm

- Psychological: hypervigilance, exaggerated startle response, irritability, sensitivity to noise, and rumination
- Behavioural: avoidance of anxiety-provoking stimuli, leading to social isolation

Phobias (F40)

The three most common phobias are agoraphobia, social phobia and simple phobia, though the boundaries between these are somewhat blurred. Note that although phobias may lead to panic attacks, a diagnosis of panic disorder excludes a diagnosis of phobia, since panic disorder is judged to be a more serious condition.

Agoraphobia (F40.0) refers to excessive worry and anxiety about being away from home, and is usually worse in situations that do not permit immediate escape such as crowded shopping areas, lifts, or public transport.

Social phobia (F40.1) describes an intense fear of being scrutinized by other people, which usually manifests itself in a fear of performing even the most mundane of activities in front of others. Those with social phobia are most often afraid of eating in front of other people.

Simple phobias (F40.2) are fears of very specific situations. Common stimuli are animals, insects, blood, dirt or contamination, heights and specific forms of travel (e.g. air travel). The latter may be difficult to distinguish from agoraphobia, though this distinction is probably of little importance.

Panic disorder (F41.0)

Discrete periods of intense fear or apprehension in which several of the symptoms of anxiety (see above) develop *suddenly* and increase in intensity over about 10 minutes. Patients characteristically believe they are in imminent danger of 'losing control'; common fears are of collapsing, having a heart attack, 'going crazy', or being incontinent. Panic attacks tend to subside within 30 minutes, and subjects may or may not experience anxiety between panic attacks. For diagnosis, the patient must have at least four panic attacks in 4 weeks, and at least four somatic symptoms must be present during each attack.

Obsessive–compulsive disorder (OCD) (F42)

Obsessions are repetitive, intrusive ideas, images and thoughts. Though unpleasant and unwanted, the subject feels that these are ego-dystonic and that resistance is impossible. The occurrence of obsessional thoughts is characteristically associated with an increase in anxiety, leading to rumination, rituals and compulsions, all of which may be viewed as means of reducing anxiety. Three-quarters of those with obsessional thoughts manifest compulsions, which frequently involve washing, cleaning and counting.

Post-traumatic stress disorder (PTSD) (F43.1)

Arises, by definition, following the experience of a traumatic event beyond the range of normal human experience, and usually involves the threat to, or loss of, life. PTSD is characterized by the persistent re-experience of the trauma, in the form of nightmares, 'flashbacks' and/or intrusive memories. Other features are depressed mood, anxiety, insomnia, poor concentration, irritability, hypervigilance and avoidance of situations that are reminiscent of the trauma.

Epidemiology

In the UK, the overall prevalence of non-psychotic psychiatric disorder in the community is approximately 16%. The most common ICD-10 diagnosis is mixed anxiety/depression, identified in nearly 8% of adults living in private households. About 2% of adults suffer from severe or moderately severe depression, and 3% from generalized anxiety disorder. About 5–6% of adults suffer from the other neurotic disorders, namely phobias, panic disorder and OCD, each of which has a prevalence of about 1%.

Basic sciences

There is evidence of a significant genetic contribution to the aetiology of the non-psychotic disorders, including depression, generalized anxiety and panic disorder. There is also evidence in favour of a common genetic risk for depression and those disorders characterized primarily by anxiety.

PET scanning studies have shown increased cerebral metabolic activity in the cingulate region and heads of the caudate nuclei and orbital gyri in individuals with OCD, as well as in related conditions such as Tourette's syndrome. It is not clear however whether obsessional thoughts are caused directly by this abnormal activity, or whether they arise indirectly, because of a failure of this dysfunctional area of cortex to filter out such thoughts. There is also evidence that OCD is associated with a relative deficiency of serotonin, since this condition responds to SSRIs (see p. 303).

Environmental factors are likely to be of aetiological importance, though the extent to which such circumstances are determined genetically remains to be determined. The clearest example of the importance of environmental influences in the pathogenesis of the neurotic disorders can be seen in PTSD, which can only arise following the experience of a severe trauma. Onset of PTSD may be delayed for several months, and the incidence among those exposed would appear to depend on subjects' pre-morbid characteristics and the severity of the trauma. This model of the pathogenesis of PTSD is consistent with extensive research documenting a causal association between threatening life events and the onset of both anxiety and depression. There is some evidence that the type of event encountered may by pathoplastic, in that anxiety is reported to follow events characterized by danger, while the onset of depression is more closely associated with events characterized by loss.

Differential diagnosis of anxiety

Organic

Alcohol or drug withdrawal/intoxication, including delirium tremens, may produce restlessness, agitation, poor concentration and subjective anxiety, apprehension or fearfulness. Anxiety and neurotic disorders are *not* associated with disorientation or fluctuations in level of consciousness. Enquire about drug and alcohol use and look for signs of drug or alcohol use. Drugs can be detected by testing urine, and liver function tests may be abnormal. Very anxious people may self-medicate with alcohol or drugs, and it may difficult to identify the primary pathology.

Thyrotoxicosis causes sweating, tachycardia, tremor and agitation. Look for signs of thyroid disease, including goitre and ophthalmic complications.

Hypoglycaemia may present with symptoms of anxiety, though onset will be acute and subject should be symptom-free except when hypoglycaemic. Enquire about history of diabetes, and check random blood glucose.

Phaeochromocytoma and carcinoid syndrome, both of which are extremely rare. In both instances anxiety, sweating, agitation, headaches and hypertension are episodic. Can test urine for VMA and 5-HIAA following 24-hour collection.

Angina/cardiac arrhythmias may present with palpitations, chest pain, and shortness of breath.

Psychiatric

- Schizophrenia may mimic OCD in particular, since unwanted experiences are (usually) perceived as ego-dystonic, and beyond voluntary control

- Mania
- Other neurotic disorder, including depression
- Dementia (see p. 192)
- Personality disorder
- Hyperventilation syndrome, a 'condition' in which individuals are highly sensitive to the somatic symptoms associated with hyperventilation (e.g. paraesthesiae), which induce high levels of anxiety, and positively reinforce this behaviour

Management

The management of depression is described on p. 210.

Although neurotic disorder is common in the community, referral to psychiatrists is rare. Most treatment is therefore provided by GPs, particularly for the more common (and less severe) disorders. In the case of mild/moderate depression and mixed anxiety/depression, there is little empirical evidence to guide treatment, and it is not known at what threshold of severity individuals benefit from antidepressant medication and what the optimum dose of this should be. Similarly, it is not known whether such individuals might derive greater benefit from psychological compared with pharmacological interventions, or whether (for example) seeing a social worker is more effective than, for example, problem solving, cognitive behavioural therapy, or psychoeducation.

More is known, however, about the treatment of the more severe anxiety disorders seen in psychiatric settings, for which first-line manage-ment usually involves behavioural and/or cog-nitive psychotherapy (see p. 324). Behavioural psychotherapy for the anxiety disorders is based on the concept of cue exposure and response prevention. The role of the therapist is to help the patient identify a graded hierarchy of fear-inducing situations, and to overcome each of these in order, beginning with the least threat-ening. In most cases, cue exposure begins with the patient imagining or talking about the situ-ation which they fear. The main goal of therapy is for the patient to tolerate exposure to the stimulus while resisting the urge to engage in the avoidance behaviour rituals for which they have sought treatment. It is necessary to explain to the patient that anxiety is a universal human experience, that intense anxiety can be tolerated without adverse effects, and that doing so will reduce both the future frequency and intensity of anxiety attacks. Such therapy may be successfully augmented by the use of relaxation techniques.

Though limited use of a benzodiazepine (alprazo-lam) is recommended (especially in the USA) evi-dence indicates that this is no more effective than behavioural psychotherapy alone, and while alprazolam alone may be as effective as behav-ioural psychotherapy initially, relapse occurs almost as soon as the medication is discontinued. Long-term benzodiazepine use is associated with dependence and a recognized withdrawal syn-drome. Caution is recommended in the prescrip-tion of benzodiazepines.

Antidepressants (especially SSRIs) and cognitive therapy may be useful as adjuvant treatments where features of depression are marked.

EATING DISORDERS I: ANOREXIA NERVOSA (ICD-10 F50.0)

Definition

Deliberate weight loss resulting in body weight less than 15% below the norm for age, sex, weight and height.

Clinical features

Behavioural

Weight loss may be achieved by many means, the most common of which are avoidance of food, overactivity and/or excessive exercise and the use of appetite suppressants, laxatives and diuretics. Self-induced vomiting is also reported, but is less prominent than in bulimia, since most anorexic individuals severely restrict their food intake. It is often the case that while anorexic individuals are rarely seen to eat, they frequently prepare food for others. As a result of their obsession with their weight and appearance, individuals suffering from anorexia weigh themselves frequently, and may spend long periods of time examining themselves in mirrors.

Physical

The predominant feature is self-induced weight loss, which frequently results in delayed puberty and/or amenorrhoea. Consequently, individuals with anorexia appear pale and emaciated, with loose-fitting clothing. Such individuals tend to have dry, thin skin and fine downy (lanugo) hair on their arms and back. The physical sequelae of anorexia nervosa are predominantly those of malnutrition. Specific physical complications include:

- Cardiovascular: bradycardia or tachycardia, hypotension, (potentially fatal) ventricular arrhythmias and/or cardiac failure. Reversible ECG abnormalities may be found

- Metabolic: impaired temperature regulation leading to hypothermia, failure of glucose metabolism leading to hypoglycaemia, hypercholesterolaemia. Repeated vomiting may cause hypokalaemia and altered blood pH

- Gastrointestinal: constipation and diarrhoea are common. Starvation leads to fatty changes in liver and hepatomegaly. Pancreatitis can occur on refeeding

- Renal: renal calculi, resulting from altered pH balance, low glomerular filtration rate and low serum Mg; may also lead to renal failure

- Haematological: pancytopenia, anaemia and bone marrow hypoplasia

- Endocrine: disturbance of sex hormone metabolism, low LH and FSH in women and low testosterone in men, impaired oogenesis and spermatogenesis, stress hormones elevated, including growth hormone and cortisol. This disturbance of the hypothalamic–pituitary–gonadal axis is responsible for amenorrhoea in women and loss of libido in men

- Skeletal: osteoporosis and/or retarded bony maturation

- Neurological: seizures

Psychological

Anorexia nervosa is characterized by a preoccupation with body weight and physical appearance. Sufferers experience a distorted body image, believing themselves to be larger (and fatter) than they are. These overvalued ideas arise in the context of a morbid fear of being fat. As a result of starvation, sleep may become disturbed with shortened REM latency, and mood may become depressed or labile. Hopelessness and suicidal thoughts may also occur.

Epidemiology

Community prevalence is believed to be about 0.5–1%, and is about 10 times higher in women compared with men. Onset is most commonly during adolescence (85% of cases). Particularly high rates of anorexia are reported among ballet dancers and models. The highest prevalence is reported in middle and upper socioeconomic groups.

The mortality associated with anorexia nervosa is of the order of 5–15%.

Basic sciences

Genetic studies indicate that MZ concordance is significantly higher than DZ concordance. The basic mechanism underlying anorexia may lie in hypothalamic dysfunction, since this is where appetite and weight are believed to be regulated. This hypothesis is supported by evidence that amenorrhoea *precedes* weight loss in 15% of cases. Structural lesions of the ventromedial part of the hypothalamus lead to starvation behaviour in animal studies. Evidence also indicates that 5-HT function may be abnormal in anorexic individuals, since 5-HT agonists produce a feeling of satiety.

Social explanations for anorexia point to the culture-specific nature of anorexia, which is not found in developing countries. Most attention has been directed towards the fashion industry in western societies and the intense social pressure for (young) women to aspire (and conform to) one particular image of female beauty.

More psychologically based theories concentrate on intrapersonal and interpersonal dynamics. Since anorexia frequently causes delayed puberty or amenorrhoea, it has been suggested that sufferers are expressing a subconscious desire to avoid (or at least to control) the emergence of an adult female sexual identity. Given the centrality of the preparation and consumption of food to family life, family theorists have suggested that anorexia, which begins in adolescence, represents an attempt at conflict resolution in families where parents are over-protective or 'enmeshed' with their children.

Differential diagnosis

Organic

- Hypopituitarism (note that in anorexia axillary and pubic hair, if established, remain intact)
- Addison's disease (note that in cases of pituitary disturbance consider space-occupying lesion)
- Thyrotoxicosis
- Inflammatory bowel disease/malabsorption (e.g. Crohn's disease or coeliac disease)

- Diabetes mellitus
- Carcinoma

Psychiatric

- Bulimia nervosa
- Depression
- OCD, which is also characterized by intrusive, unwanted, repetitive, anxiety-provoking thoughts. Indeed, since anorexic individuals have a morbid fear of losing control over the appearance of their bodies it has been suggested that anorexia is a variant on OCD. It is possible that both may be mediated by abnormalities in 5-HT transmission.

Management

The main aim of treatment is the restoration of a healthy weight and healthy eating habits. This is best achieved gradually, and success depends on the establishment of a therapeutic alliance with the patient. Since the primary pathology appears to lie in the patient's fear of losing control over their body, it is crucial that they be helped to understand the importance of a healthy weight, and that they gradually assume responsibility for achieving and maintaining this. It must be stressed that it is possible for the patient to gain weight without losing control over their body.

Hospital admission may be necessary if weight loss is rapid or severe (<25% of ideal body weight). Other indications for admission are hypokalaemia or other serious metabolic disturbance, severe depression and/or suicidal ideation, and cycles of starvation and/or binge eating that cannot be interrupted by means of outpatient treatment. Inpatient treatment depends on high-quality nursing care, and comprises bed-rest, restriction of activities and a diet of 3000–5000 kcal per day. The most commonly adopted approach is based on a behavioural model, in which weight gain is rewarded by increasing mobility and privileges. This regimen should result in a weight gain of 1.0–1.5 kg per week. If weight loss is life-threatening it may be necessary to introduce parenteral nutrition, under the terms of the Mental Health Act.

The most effective long-term treatment for anorexia nervosa is probably cognitive behavioural therapy, further emphasizing the connection between this condition and the neurotic disorders. The aim of such treatment is to identify (and remedy) the dysfunctional cognitions associated with self-starvation or binge eating, including low self-esteem, feelings of powerlessness, and perfectionist tendencies. Family therapy has also proved effective, and is particularly helpful when the patient is an adolescent living with their parents. The aim is to understand the role that the illness plays in family life, and to help the family towards less destructive means of conflict resolution.

EATING DISORDERS II: BULIMIA NERVOSA (ICD-10 F50.2)

Bulimia is an eating disorder closely associated with anorexia nervosa, and which may follow the onset of anorexia chronologically. While the psychopathological features of bulimia resemble those of anorexia, bulimia differs from anorexia in that weight is either normal or increased.

Definition

Bulimia nervosa is characterized by repeated bouts of overeating and an excessive preoccupation with the control of body weight.

Clinical features

Bulimia is characterized by binge eating, followed by purging, usually in the form of self-induced vomiting. Bulimia represents a (near-) complete loss of control over eating, and it has been said that while anorexic individuals may go for long periods without experiencing hunger, bulimic individuals experience an intense craving for food. Thus, sufferers from bulimia attempt to control their weight through a variety of methods, of which vomiting and purging with laxatives or diuretics are the most common.

Episodes of bingeing and purging may be precipitated by feelings of depression, anxiety, boredom or loneliness. During binges large quantities of (typically) carbohydrate-rich food are consumed rapidly with little attention to taste. Foods selected for binges are those which the individual perceives as forbidden (e.g. chocolate bars, cakes and biscuits) and which they usually deny themselves. As many as 10 000 kcal may be consumed in a single episode, which is usually followed by feelings of intense guilt and self-loathing.

Though both anorexia and bulimia occur among individuals with low self-esteem who perceive themselves as powerless, those with bulimia may be more likely to engage in other forms of self-injurious behaviour (e.g. overdoses).

The physical sequelae of bulimia differ markedly from those of anorexia, in that the stigmata are those associated with purging rather than starvation. Principal among these are:

- Salivary gland enlargement
- Erosion of dental enamel
- Calluses on the dorsum of the hand (Russell's sign)
- Metabolic disturbances, especially alkalosis and hypokalaemia

Epidemiology

The best available estimate is that the prevalence of bulimia is similar to that of anorexia, namely 0.5–1%. It is estimated that about half of those meeting criteria for bulimia would have met criteria for anorexia nervosa in the past. Like anorexia, bulimia is most prevalent among women and in higher socioeconomic groups. It is believed that the peak age of onset of bulimia is in the 20s, slightly later than anorexia.

Basic science

Given the similarity of their age and sex distribution, and the common psychopathology, it is likely that bulimia and anorexia are also aetiologically similar. The primary difference between these conditions is that bulimic individuals experience far greater urges to eat than anorexic individuals. It is possible, therefore, that the patterns of neurotransmitter dysfunction underlying these two conditions may differ to an extent. Thus, anorexic individuals appear to have less difficulty in controlling their appetites than bulimic individuals, who cope with their psychopathology by purging themselves.

Differential diagnosis

- Upper gastrointestinal disorders, which cause repeated vomiting, e.g. duodenal ulcer
- Depression
- Personality disorder, particularly borderline type (ICD-10 F60.31)

Management

Since bulimia is rarely a life-threatening condition, the overwhelming majority of patients may be managed as outpatients. Admission may be indicated, however, if the patient is severely depressed, at risk of suicide, or if they are suffering from severe physical ill-health as a result of bingeing and purging. In certain instances it may also be helpful to admit patients whose illness proves resistant to outpatient treatment.

There is limited evidence that some patients may benefit from SSRI antidepressants, such as fluvoxamine and fluoxetine.

The mainstay of treatment is cognitive behaviour therapy, through which patients' eating habits and attitudes about their weight and physical appearance may be modified.

DISORDERS OF PERSONALITY
(ICD-10 F60-69)

The concept of personality disorder as a diagnostic entity has arisen out of attempts to classify a variety of dysfunctional behaviours that are often poorly understood, and which are largely unresponsive to treatment. While psychologists have preferred to conceptualize personality in terms of a variety of continuously distributed traits, psychiatrists have traditionally opted instead for categorical models.

Personality disorders therefore represent persistent and characteristic patterns of behaviour and ways of relating to the self and others. Central to the definition of personality disorder is the notion that these behaviours are harmful to the individual or others.

Definition

Enduring maladaptive patterns of behaviour, modes of thinking and relating to oneself, the environment and others which cause either impairment in social functioning or considerable distress to the individual or others. These personality features should be recognizable by adolescence, and should persist throughout adult life. Personality disorders are primary and not secondary to other psychiatric or physical disorders.

Within ICD-10, personality disorders correspond to clusters of traits. A diagnosis of personality disorder should only be made on the basis of more than one interview with the patient, and with information from as many informants as possible. Eight specific personality disorders are listed in ICD-10.

Clinical features

Paranoid personality disorder (F60.0)

Excessive sensitivity to setbacks, a tendency to bear grudges and harbour resentments, suspiciousness, unwillingness to trust others, litigiousness and a preoccupation with 'conspiracy theories'. Individuals with paranoid personality disorder often suspect their spouse or partner of being unfaithful, and have a tendency towards self-importance. Such individuals are extremely 'brittle' and, contrary to their protestations, have an extremely fragile self-esteem, which they are required to bolster continuously by means of projection.

Schizoid personality disorder (F60.1)

Cold and aloof, these individuals do not appear to take pleasure from any activities and seem incapable of expressing strong positive or negative emotions. Affect cold, detached or flat. Little capacity for, or interest in, intimate relationships (including sexual relationships). Thus, individuals with schizoid personality disorder have few friends and appear to prefer solitary pursuits. Social awkwardness may be very prominent. A further defining characteristic is an apparent insensitivity to praise or criticism.

Dissocial personality disorder (F60.2)

Perhaps the most dangerous of all the personality disorders, characterized by antisocial behaviour and callous disregard for the feelings, safety and well-being of others. Dissocial personality disorder incorporates the earlier categories of sociopathic and psychopathic personality disorders.

Those with dissocial personality disorder are irresponsible, show no concern for rules or social norms, and are often in conflict with authority. There is a characteristic inability to tolerate frustration, resulting in aggressive and violent behaviour. Individuals with dissocial personality disorder appear incapable of experiencing remorse and tend to blame others (including their victims) for their own shortcomings and misdeeds. There is some empirical evidence that such individuals are incapable of learning from punishment or rewards, which may reflect underlying brain dysfunction.

Emotionally unstable personality disorder (F60.3)

Two types of emotionally unstable personality disorder are listed in ICD-10, *impulsive type* (F60.30) and *borderline type* (F60.31). Both are characterized by emotional instability, poor self-control and impulsive behaviour. Emotions are experienced with unbearable intensity, leading to explosive outbursts and attempts at self-harm. In the impulsive form of this personality disorder individuals respond to criticism with violent or threatening outbursts. Individuals with borderline personality disorder are said to have a 'chronic sense of emptiness', and may become involved in intense and unstable personal relationships. Emotional crises are common, often arising out of a fear of abandonment. Such individuals may experience transient psychotic episodes, such is the intensity of their emotions. Some individuals with borderline personality disorder cope with their unbearable internal feelings by indulging in self-mutilating behaviours such as cutting or burning their arms or legs, while others may take overdoses or make more serious attempts at suicide. The cardinal feature of self-mutilating behaviour in borderline personality disorder is that the patient reports an immediate release of anxiety on inflicting the wound.

Histrionic personality disorder (F60.4)

Self-dramatizing and theatrical behaviour, often perceived by others as attention-seeking. Shallow, labile affect. Individuals with histrionic personality disorder seek excitement, and gain a reputation for melodrama. They appear vain, egotistical and self-absorbed, and are largely incapable of forming enduring close relationships or showing genuine concern for others. A characteristic scenario is that in which the support of friends or family is enlisted in dealing with a crisis that never materializes or which turns out to be rather trivial. The individual with histrionic personality disorder then moves on to the next 'crisis' without apparent concern for the distress this may cause others. As a result such individuals often alienate those nearest to them, gaining a reputation for 'crying wolf'.

Anankastic personality disorder (F60.5)

Characterized by caution, anxiety and self-doubt, such individuals are thought to be 'obsessional', appearing preoccupied with order and the observation of rules. The archetypal 'perfectionist', a trait which ceases to be of benefit to the individual but instead leads to a paralysing rigidity in the approach to any task. The same applies to tidiness, conscientiousness, and scrupulous: though assets in moderation, these traits are extremely damaging in their extreme forms. The anankastic individual is therefore pedantic and stubborn, to an extent that precludes compromise and thus close relationships with others.

Anxious (avoidant) personality disorder (F60.6)

Characterized by constant feelings of apprehension and low self-esteem, exacerbated by fear of social inadequacy. Fear of humiliation or rejection in social interactions, and therefore an avoidance of other people. Hypersensitive to criticism.

Dependent personality disorder (F60.7)

Such individuals are unwilling to take responsibility for important decisions in their lives, preferring for others to make these. Passivity, and acquiescence to those on whom they depend is characteristic, as are feelings of helplessness when alone. Dependent individuals require enormous reassurance when making even the simplest independent decisions.

Epidemiology

Almost impossible to estimate the prevalence of most personality disorders, since there have been no community-based epidemiological studies.

Basic science

Most aetiological enquiry in the field of personality disorders has focused on dissocial personality disorder (psychopathy), a syndrome that rarely occurs in the absence of a history of childhood antisocial behaviour. Such individuals often come from disturbed homes, and associations have been reported with a paternal history of antisocial behaviour as well as childhood physical and/or sexual abuse. Such findings are consistent with both biological (genetic) and environmental models.

Genetic studies have estimated concordance rates for MZ twins at 36% and for DZ twins at 12%, suggesting a strong genetic contribution to psychopathy.

There is also evidence of abnormal brain function among psychopaths. One well-known finding is that widespread slow waves are seen on the EEGs of up to 60% of individuals diagnosed as psychopathic. This neurophysiological abnormality appears to be more common among psychopaths with a history of aggressive or violent behaviour. It has been suggested that the inability of psychopaths to learn from noxious experiences (e.g. punishment) reflects cortical immaturity or minimal brain damage. The frontal and temporal lobes appear to be the most likely site of any focal abnormality.

Differential diagnosis

The differential diagnosis will vary for different specific personality disorders. Although other psychiatric disorders can occur in the context of an abnormal or dysfunctional personality, it is usual to diagnose a personality disorder only in the absence of an alternative psychiatric diagnosis. In view of the stigma attached to 'personality disorder' this diagnosis should be made cautiously, and with great care.

Thus, other major psychiatric disorders

should be excluded before a diagnosis of personality disorder is made. The following should be considered:

- Schizophrenia (note that the negative symptoms of chronic schizophrenia can appear as apathy, passivity or dependence)
- Mania can mimic histrionic personality disorder
- Depression
- Generalized anxiety disorder/panic disorder/social phobia
- OCD
- Somatoform/dissociative disorders
- Drug and/or alcohol dependency
- Anorexia nervosa or bulimia nervosa

Management

Since the defining feature of personality disorders is that they represent 'enduring maladaptive patterns of behaviour', prognosis is usually poor. It is therefore essential that treatment of such individuals is pragmatic. In general there is little likelihood of significant change in personality, although over longer periods of time dysfunctional behaviours may be modifiable.

Few individuals with personality disorder enter into psychiatric treatment, and those that do are likely to be referred because of antisocial behaviour or severe difficulties in social functioning.

The dysfunctional behaviours that cause so much distress reflect interactions between the individual with personality disorder and his or her environment. Since personality is likely to be resistant to change, it is often much more productive and helpful to identify aspects of the patient's environment which might be modified. Thus, individuals with personality disorder can be advised to structure their lives (e.g. in terms of accommodation, occupation and social contacts) in such a way as to minimize conflict and psychological distress. Thus, the mainstay of treatment for most individuals with personality disorders is low-intensity supportive psychotherapy, combined with supervision of those individuals at risk of antisocial behaviour.

Though it has been suggested that some patients with personality disorder may benefit from long-term psychoanalytic psychotherapy there is little empirical evidence to support the effectiveness of such treatment.

The Mental Health Act, 1983 makes provision for the formal (compulsory) treatment of just one type of personality disorder, psychopathy. Though most psychiatrists believe such individuals to be resistant to treatment, this aspect of the Mental Health Act allows for individuals with dissocial personality disorder to be detained in psychiatric hospital (e.g. special hospitals) for the protection of others.

Learning Difficulties (ICD-10 F70–79)

Definition

There has been considerable debate in recent years over the most appropriate nomenclature for this group of disorders, which have been referred to in the past as imbecility, feeble-mindedness, mental subnormality, mental deficiency, mental retardation and mental handicap as well as learning disability and learning difficulties. Though 'learning difficulties' is generally preferred by health professionals, users and carers in the UK, ICD-10 classifies these conditions under the general heading of 'mental retardation'.

According to ICD-10 mental retardation is defined as a condition of *incomplete* mental development, as distinct from a *deterioration* in psychological or social functioning (as in dementia). The cardinal feature of mental retardation is 'a reduced level of intellectual functioning resulting in a diminished ability to adapt to the daily demands of the normal social environment'. Mental retardation is therefore characterized by deficits in motor, cognitive, linguistic and social skills compared with population norms. The clinical features of these disorders must also be present before adulthood.

ICD-10 subdivides the continuum of impaired intellectual functioning into four categories of mental retardation: mild (F70), moderate (F71), severe (F72) and profound (F73).

Clinical features

A definite diagnosis of mental retardation requires evidence of a reduced level of intellectual functioning compared with the appropriate population norm. Although it is tempting to make this judgement solely on the basis of IQ score, it must be remembered that intelligence is not a unitary construct. Thus, there may be significant discrepancies between skill levels in different domains of functioning. The assessment of intellectual functioning should be based on as many sources of information as possible, and should involve formal psychometric testing including standardized, individually administered IQ tests. According to ICD-10, only a provisional diagnosis is permissible in the absence of standardized assessment procedures.

Mild mental retardation (F70) (IQ 50–69)

Characterized by delay in skill acquisition. Most mildly retarded individuals are able to function at a sufficient level to achieve full independence as adults, including eating and self-care (washing, dressing and toileting). Though conversational language is usually satisfactory, academic school work is usually significantly below average, with particular deficits in reading and writing. Individuals with mild mental retardation are often capable of maintaining semi-skilled employment that requires practical abilities but not written language skills. Social and emotional handicaps may or may not be overtly noticeable.

Moderate mental retardation (F71) (IQ 35–49)

Marked delay in the acquisition of language skills, with limited eventual achievement in this area. Achievement of other skills, notably self-care, is also impaired. Acquisition of language skills is variable. While academic school work is significantly below normal, many may acquire basic literacy skills. As adults, moderately mentally retarded individuals are able to do simple practical tasks, though these usually need to be highly structured. Complete independent living is rarely achieved. Though fully mobile, interpersonal social skills may be grossly limited. Discrepant profiles of abilities are common.

Severe mental retardation (F72) (IQ 20–34)

Similar clinical picture to that observed in moderate mental retardation, though with generally lower levels of social and intellectual functioning. Most people in this category also suffer from impaired motor function, indicating significant damage or maldevelopment of the CNS (e.g. spasticity and athetosis).

Profound mental retardation (F73) (IQ less than 20)

Affected individuals are severely limited in their ability to comprehend and use language. Most are also immobile, incontinent and capable of little more than rudimentary non-verbal communication. Profoundly mentally retarded individuals are rarely able to perform any of the tasks involved in self-care, and therefore require continuous supervision.

Epidemiology

Level	IQ	Proportion of population	Proportion of those with mental retardation
Mild	50–69	1.5%	80%
Moderate	35–49	0.3%	12%
Severe	20–34	0.2%	7%
Profound	<20	0.05%	1%

Although IQ test scoring is based on the assumption that intelligence is normally distributed, there are more people in the UK with an IQ below 70 than predicted on the basis of the normal distribution. The slight degree of skewing at the lower end of the IQ distribution is probably due to the occurrence of pathological causes of low IQ (i.e. genetic causes) superimposed on a normally distributed characteristic in the general population.

Learning difficulties are more common in males, probably as a result of genetic abnormalities associated with the X chromosome. The prevalence of other psychiatric disorders (including the psychoses) is three to four times greater among individuals with learning difficulties than in the general population.

Epilepsy, and physical and neurological disabilities are very common in those with moderate, severe and profound mental retardation, and the size of association may well be directly related to the severity of intellectual impairment.

Basic sciences

In mild mental retardation there are no specific causes usually; these people represent the lower range of IQ distribution within the population. Where there is more than just mild deficits, there is often an organic cause. The most common of these are:

- Chromosomal abnormalities: e.g. X-linked syndromes such as fragile X syndrome, Turner's syndrome, Klinefelter's syndrome and Down's syndrome, which affects 1/1000 live births

- Genetic abnormalities: e.g. phenylketonuria, homocystinuria, Tay–Sachs disease, Lesch–Nyhan disease, tuberous sclerosis, Niemann–Pick disease, Hurler's disease and neurofibromatosis

- Intrauterine infection: cytomegalovirus, rubella, syphilis, toxoplasmosis
- Intrauterine insult: fetal alcohol syndrome, heavy metal poisoning or teratogenic drugs
- Endocrine disorders: hypothyroidism
- Neonatal trauma: hypoxia or intraventricular haemorrhage from various causes, more common in premature delivery (cerebral palsy)
- Cranial malformations: hydrocephalus
- Childhood infection: meningitis, encephalitis
- Childhood head injury

It is known from Rutter's work in the Isle of Wight that children who are of normal intelligence and brain damaged are more likely to have psychiatric disorders. Epilepsy is especially linked to developmental abnormalities and low IQ. Furthermore repeated seizures have been hypothesized to further damage neuronal tissue although damaged tissue is often the focus of seizures also.

Differential diagnosis

Those with learning difficulties can develop all the range of mental illnesses described elsewhere. Hence one should consider the main groups of disorders but the assessment is usually complex and requires a careful appraisal of the context in which disturbed behaviour is displayed as superficially similar behaviours after careful exploration might be attributable to hallucinosis or frustration in a depressed patient. A specialist team should be consulted. Assess physical impairments and sensory deficits. Many apparently unusual behaviours may be related to the difficult negotiation of development stages, perhaps to do with individuation, intimate sexual relationships and family relationships. Assessment is especially compromised when the IQ is less than 50 such that communication is impaired. In this instance assessment and management are based on any identifiable phenomenon.[1]

Management

The most important point to bear in mind is that there are three aspects of the problems experienced by patients: the impairment itself (e.g. organic brain damage), the disability (e.g. illiteracy) and the social handicap arising from the disability.

While it is essential to try to identify the source of the impairment, by means of careful assessment, it is probably more important to consider the current needs of the patient and his/her carers. A careful developmental history should be undertaken, including all childhood investigations with an outline of varying functional abilities and associated environmental and mental state findings. Family assessment is also essential.

PSYCHOLOGICAL

In the absence of effective communication a behavioural analysis should be carried out, focusing on problem behaviours, their antecedents and consequences. It may be that it is only from the behaviour that one can ascertain the underlying mental state. Supportive counselling and frank discussion with a trusted professional are invaluable to aid assessment and enable the patient to get a better understanding and develop coping strategies. Family work is also important especially after diagnosis, or when the presentation changes and places the family in crisis also.

BIOLOGICAL

Drug treatments are often used to control behaviour. These treatments are sometimes used without a good assessment of the underlying mental state. The response to medication is then often, in error perhaps, used to support a diagnosis. The safest antipsychotic to use is haloperidol. Benzodiazepines are also used acutely, but for mood stabilization, irritability and manic states lithium and carbamezepine are used to good effect. Lithium is also used to control unexplained states of self-mutilation and frustration leading to tantrums. Propranolol and clonidine also have been used to control self-destructive behaviours. Where there are specific symptoms of depression or where behaviour (e.g. crying, withdrawal) indicate depression antidepressants should be prescribed.

SOCIAL

This involves the provision of support for families if the patient is still living with parents and/or sibs. More usually it is necessary to ensure that an adequate level of supported housing is available. Those with major mental illness will need specialist supported housing where the staff are familiar with caring for the mentally ill as well as working and living with those with learning difficulties. Places of work and leisure are also necessary as part of an overall rehabilitation package.

CHILD AND ADOLESCENT PSYCHIATRY

General principles

Child and adolescent psychiatrists work within the context of a multidisciplinary team from child guidance centres and specialist departments. A child presenting with difficulties is always assessed within a developmental context, and is assessed as part of a larger system: the child's family, culture, educational establishment and social network. Much of the therapeutic work with children is offered via this system, and though assessment and treatment may take place at a central location, therapeutic interventions may take place in the child's home or school. Liaison tends to take place to a great degree with both educational facilities and social services. Though inpatient units exist where both individuals and families can be treated, the vast majority of therapeutic interventions take place on an outpatient basis or in the community. Therefore in many ways the established pattern of service delivery in child and adolescent psychiatry is a blueprint for the newer community adult services currently in development.

In terms of treatment, the use of psychotropic drugs in child psychiatry is generally uncommon in the UK. Family therapy, school liaison, supportive therapy with the child, and behavioural interventions are the more common treatment modalities.

Presentation

There are four main patterns of presenting symptomatology: disturbances in conduct, emotions, relationships or development delay(s). A disturbed child rarely presents him or herself for assessment: the disturbance has usually become apparent to others, typically parents, teachers, or the police in the case of juvenile offenders. If the referral was suggested by someone else, the parents may initially be hostile. Consequently, the presenting problems always need to be viewed as a disturbance resting not solely in the child, but also within the concerned carers.

Diagnosis

In considering whether a child may have a psychiatric disorder, an important principle is that both symptoms and handicap (social incapacity) are assessed. A developmental and thorough family history is usually taken from parents, and supplementary sources are used for a history of current difficulties to assess whether the child's disturbance is apparent in only one situation or is generalized. This information is used as the basis for an interview with, and examination of, the child. Psychological testing may be warranted to determine intelligence, educational achievements, personality assessment and motor and perceptual development. Often the child is observed within the context of a family interview or a structured play setting with his or her family members. There are important issues around confidentiality in this assessment procedure, in that information that puts a child at risk may need to be shared with other professionals.

A multi-axial diagnosis (proposed originally by Rutter) is used in many centres to take account of the wider context and is reflected in ICD-10 codings.

Axis I	Clinical psychiatric syndromes
00–09	Organic mental disorders
10–19	Mental and behavioural disorders due to psychoactive substance use
20–29	Schizophrenia, schizotypal and delusional disorders
30–39	Mood (affective) disorders
40–48	Neurotic, stress-related and somatoform disorders
50–59	Behavioural syndromes associated with physiological disturbances and physical factors
60–69	Disorders of personality and behaviour
84	Pervasive developmental disorders
90–98	Behavioural and emotional disorders with onset usually occurring in childhood or adolescence
99	Unspecified mental disorder

Axis II	Specific disorders of psychological development
80	Specific developmental disorders of speech and language
81	Specific developmental disorders of scholastic skills
82	Specific developmental disorder of motor function
83	Mixed specific developmental disorders
88	Other disorders of psychological development
89	Unspecified disorder of psychological development

Axis III	Intellectual level
70	Mild mental retardation
71	Moderate mental retardation
72	Severe mental retardation
73	Profound mental retardation
78	Other mental retardation

79   Unspecified mental retardation

Axis IV   Medical conditions

**Axis V   Associated abnormal
            psychosocial situations**
01   Abnormal intrafamilial relationships
02   Mental disorder, deviance or
            handicap in the child's primary
            support group
03   Inadequate or distorted intrafamilial
            communication
04   Abnormal qualities of upbringing
05   Abnormal immediate environment
06   Acute life events
07   Societal stressors
08   Chronic interpersonal stress
            associated with school work
09   Stressful events/situations resulting
            from child's own disorder/disability

**Axis VI   Global assessment of
            psychosocial disability**
0   Superior/good social functioning
graded to
8   Profound and pervasive social disability

Specific diagnoses

In this section attention is paid to common disorders where the presentation may differ from
that of an adult, and to the specific syndromes
that manifest solely or usually in childhood or
adolescence.

Emotional disorders

Depression Epidemiological   studies   show
that many children are miserable. In the Isle of

Wight studies, about 10% of 10 year olds were miserable according to their parents, and over 40% of 14 year olds were miserable by their own account. Depression presents in different ways at different developmental stages: pre-school children often experience despair if separated from their attachment figures. From about the age of 6 years, the phenomenology of depressive disorders begins to resemble that of adult depression, and similar diagnostic criteria are therefore applied. In childhood, depression may present as school refusal, friendship difficulties, irritability, and somatic complaints. Suicidal thoughts can occur in quite young children, but plans do not usually become potentially fatal until adolescence. The sex ratio for childhood depression is equal, with the adult female preponderance becoming evident in adolescence. Half of depressed children have at least one other psychiatric disorder, typically conduct or anxiety disorders.

The role of medication in treatment is controversial. Its use is more common in post-pubertal children. Cognitive therapy is becoming more widely used, in addition to family and individual therapy and school liaison.

Mania Classical mania is rare in childhood. An important differential diagnosis is a hyperkinetic disorder. Mania in adolescence is commonly misdiagnosed as schizophrenia as first rank symptoms are often prominent.

Anxiety disorders Between 5 and 10% of children and adolescents may have clinically significant anxiety disorders. The three commonest are separation anxiety disorder (fear of separation, arising in early childhood, of an unusual severity, persisting to a developmentally inappropriate extent, associated with significant social dysfunction), simple phobias and generalized anxiety disorder. Anxiety disorders may present as school refusal, somatic disorders, poor self-confidence and poor school performance.

School attendance problems are relatively common in any childhood emotional disorder, and may also be caused by bullying and difficulties with scholastic achievement. The child may complain of headache or abdominal pain on school mornings. A mother can covertly encourage the child if she herself is reluctant to be separated from the child or has emotional or other problems. Treatment involves rapidly re-establishing a pattern of school attendance, often supportive therapy for the child and mother, and dealing with any contributory problems at the school.

Conduct disorders

ICD-10 defines these as 'disorders characterised by a repetitive and persistent pattern of dissocial, aggressive, or defiant conduct'. The antisocial conduct may include lying, stealing, truancy, fire-setting, cruelty to animals and vandalism. The behaviour pattern needs to be enduring, i.e. of 6 months or longer, and should be more severe than expected for the developmental level of the child. Conduct disorders are associated with underlying brain damage, adverse social circumstances, and a family pattern of harsh and inconsistent discipline with poor monitoring and little child-centred activity. Antisocial behaviour in children may be a developmental trait starting with temper tantrums and possibly leading to criminality, alcoholism, unemployment and marital discord later in life.

Conduct disorder can be classified as:

- Confined to the family context
- Unsocialized: associated with significant pervasive abnormalities in the individual's relationships with other children
- Socialized: occurring in individuals who are generally well integrated into their peer group
- Oppositional defiant: usually in younger children with defiant, disobedient behaviour that does not usually include delinquent acts
- Other/unspecified

Mixed conduct and emotional disorders are relatively common.

Treatment for conduct disorders involves family therapy, which may either be based on modification of the child's behaviours or focus on parent–child interactions. It is often combined with social casework.

Relationship disorders

Sibling rivalry disorder is an unusual degree or persistence of emotional disturbance following the birth of a younger sibling.

Elective mutism is an emotionally determined selectivity in speaking often associated with social anxiety, withdrawal, sensitivity or resistance.

Reactive attachment disorder involves persistent abnormalities in the child's pattern of social relationships associated with emotional disturbance and reactive to changes in environmental circumstances. The syndrome often results from severe parental neglect or abuse.

Disinhibited attachment disorder consists of diffuse non-selective attachment behaviour, attention-seeking and indiscriminate friendly behaviour, sometimes with poorly modulated peer interactions, and persisting beyond a developmentally appropriate age.

Developmental disorders

Pervasive developmental disorders are characterized by qualitative abnormalities in reciprocal social interactions and in patterns of communication, and by a restricted, stereotyped, repetitive repertoire of interests and activities. These features are present in all situations.

Childhood autism is generally believed to be a genetically influenced neurodevelopmental disorder defined by abnormal or impaired development present before the age of 3 years and with characteristic abnormalities in communication, social interaction and restricted repetitive behaviours. Atypical autism is marked either by a later onset or abnormal functioning in only two of the three domains.

Rett's syndrome occurs in girls with apparently normal early development followed by partial or complete loss of speech and skills in locomotion and hand use.

Other childhood disintegrative disorders also show a period of apparently normal development followed by loss of skills in several areas of development.

Asperger's syndrome is characterized by abnormalities in reciprocal social interaction with restricted or stereotyped interests, but in the context of normal language and cognitive development. It may be associated with clumsiness and there is a strong tendency towards depression in later life.

Specific disorders of psychological development are coded on Axis II and include articulation disorder, expressive and receptive language disorders, specific reading, spelling and arithmetic disorders (including dyslexia) and specific developmental disorder of motor function.

Other psychiatric disorders seen in children and adolescents

Hyperkinetic disorders are believed to be of neurodevelopmental aetiology and are characterized by early onset, lack of persistence in activities that require cognitive involvement, and a tendency to move from one activity to another without completing any one. Activity is often excessive and disorganized, and affected children may be accident-prone, reckless, and often form socially disinhibited relationships with adults. Disciplinary problems are common, as are difficulties in motor and language development and scholastic skills. Hyperkinetic disorders are more common in boys, and may be associated with aggression, mild mental handicap, epilepsy and minor motor abnormalities. Treatment is usually by behavioural modification with special teaching methods. Careful use of a cerebral stimulant, such as methylphenidate, may bring relief to the level of a child being able to concentrate at school. Side-effects include appetite suppression, stunted growth and addiction and therefore monitoring must be ongoing and careful.

Substance misuse is relatively frequent and includes glue-sniffing, tobacco and alcohol consumption, and use of illicit substances such as marijuana, cocaine crack and ecstasy. Peer and cultural pressures play an important part in establishing a pattern of substance misuse and educational programmes are designed to raise awareness in teachers and parents of the symptoms and signs of intoxication, and to educate youngsters on the detrimental effects of such substances. Substance misuse is more common in children with a history of conduct disorder.

Eating disorders often have an onset in adolescence and are dealt with more fully on p. 239. Family therapy is usually the treatment of choice in anorexia.

Psychoses including schizophrenia can present in childhood but more commonly in adolescence. Lack of acute inpatient facilities for young adolescents is a nationwide problem. Initial presentation can be insidious, with gradual deterioration in functioning at school and in peer relationships, or very florid, where a differential diagnosis of substance misuse is often considered. Issues such as living in a family with hgh expressed emotion are particularly important in adolescent schizophrenia.

Obsessive–compulsive disorder can have an early onset, particularly with obsessive ruminations or obsessive neatness.

Adjustment disorders and post-traumatic stress disorder are relatively frequent and may go undiagnosed, particularly after a bereavement where the child may have been 'protected' by not being invited to attend the funeral or to talk about his or her feelings around the death of a relative, leading to delayed or abnormal mourning. Death of a parent or divorce will also involve disruptions to caring, possibly a move of home or school, and can result in significant emotional disturbance.

Sleep disorders with onset in childhood include sleepwalking, sleep terrors and nightmares. Sleepwalking usually occurs during the first third of sleep, involves low levels of awareness and reactivity, and there is no recall of the event upon waking. Sleep terrors are very worrying to parents, involving terror, vocalization and motility. They usually occur in the first third of sleep and recall on waking is very limited.

Trichotillomania occurs more commonly in girls and involves pulling out hairs as a result of mounting tension. Treatment addresses the underlying anxiety and is often cognitive/behavioural in orientation.

Tic disorders involve involuntary, rapid, recurrent, non-rhythmic motor movements or vocal production. Gilles de la Tourette's syndrome is the most severe manifestation comprising multiple tics and compulsive utterances. Treatment with haloperidol and behavioural interventions may be effective.

Enuresis is involuntary voiding of urine that is abnormal in relation to the individual's mental age and not secondary to an organic problem. A behavioural regimen is often used in treatment involving star charts and bell-and-pad mechanisms. Use of tricyclic antidepressants may be successful for short critical periods such as family holidays.

Encopresis is voluntary or involuntary passage of faeces in inappropriate places. It can occur monosymptomatically or as part of a wider disorder of emotions or conduct. Treatment involves ruling out an organic cause, addressing underlying disturbance and behavioural management.

Special problems in child and adolescent psychiatry

Child abuse

Child abuse is an increasingly recognized problem and may be physical, sexual or emotional in nature. Most child abuse is carried out by parents or close relatives/carers. Such parents often have a history of being abused themselves and are often socially disadvantaged. Children who are handicapped in some way are more likely to be abused. Abuse of any form may present as withdrawal, fearfulness, as an emotional or conduct disorder or as poor functioning at school.

Physical abuse, or non-accidental injury, may present as broken bones, retinal haemorrhage or cigarette burns. The child may be retarded in mental, physical or social development. Sexual abuse is concealed and children are coerced into secrecy with threats. Most victims are girls where their assailants are usually known to them. Boys are abused more commonly by strangers or persons in authority. The presentation is often indirect, such as by running away from home, emotional or schooling difficulties, or genital infection. Cases of child sexual abuse may not present until adulthood, underlying self-harm behaviour, psychosexual difficulties, or emotional or personality disorders.

Emotional abuse includes parenting patterns of neglect, and being habitually critical and rejecting, and the child may present with developmental delay or disordered behaviour.

If a doctor suspects abuse he or she is normally required by the GMC to disclose to a statutory agency such as social services, the NSPCC or the police. The Area Child Protection Committee will have a policy on who has responsibility for convening conferences – preliminary consultation to test the professional hypothesis, strategy discussions, and child protection conferences. The Children's Act, 1989 outlines the procedures to be followed in suspected abuse cases. The main principles are:

- The child's welfare is paramount
- Parents have responsibilities to their children and have to be kept informed about their children and participate in decision making
- Wherever possible children should be cared for within their own families
- Children should also be kept informed and participate in decision making about their future
- With regard to the Court, an order for care under the Act should only be made if it would be better for the child than making no order at all; any delay in proceedings is likely to prejudice the child's welfare; in disputed cases the Court must have regard for the child's wishes and feelings

Deliberate self-harm

Deliberate self-harm and suicide attempts are relatively common in adolescence, particularly amongst girls. Casualty officers may need to be aware of particular factors. Repeated wrist-slashing appears to be more common in those who have been abused as children and is often associated with a multi-impulsive disorder involving eating disorders, alcohol and substance abuse, and reckless sexual activity. Drug overdoses may be a reaction to relationship problems and, though often attention-seeking, may be serious because of lack of awareness of the potential dangers of over-the-counter medications especially paracetamol. Sometimes outbreaks of copy-cat behaviour result in increased self-harm attempts within a peer group or as a result of media focus on the suicide attempt of a soap-opera or real-life star. Ideally all young people making a suicide attempt should be assessed by a child psychiatrist within the context of their family, and in most areas this is a requirement in cases of repeated attempts.

OTHER BEHAVIOURAL DISORDERS

Puerperal disorders

Although listed under this section within the ICD-10 classification, these disorders are discussed on p. 126.

Sexual problems

Sexual problems amongst the mentally ill have become of greater concern for several reasons.

- The mentally ill, despite disabilities, do have active sex lives but recent concerns about HIV have raised the possibility that they may not be informed about safe sex.

- Mental illness and sexual functioning have several interfaces: a confiding relationship is a protective factor for women with depression; expressed emotions invariably arise in the context of a relationship, of which sexual matters are one aspect; mental illness vulnerability factors may be of aetiological significance in sexual and relationship problems amongst the mentally ill and those presenting to sex and marital therapy clinics; drugs used for the treatment of mental illness interfere with sexual functioning. Furthermore those with sexual and/or relationship problems may develop anxiety and depressive states and hence present to the psychiatrist or need psychiatric intervention in the course of sexual and marital therapy.

- The mentally ill are the target of concerns from the public and professionals about inappropriate sexual displays, which can range from clumsy and naive sexual exploration to potentially assaultative behaviour.

- Underlying these concerns is the greater public profile of mentally ill patients since the larger institutions have closed.

Assessment

Sexual arousal arises from several components that are truly psychosomatic in terms of their interaction. Arousal usually involves a cognitive component involving a desire to have sexual relations, sexual fantasy or visualization, tactile sensations from skin, other influences such as the smell of perfumes, and the physiological responses indicating arousal and enabling sexual intercourse; these can interact in any order and some may be more important than others to specific individuals. An assessment should be directed to each of these. The main concern is that many physical illnesses can also have an adverse effect on sexual functioning and these should be excluded by obtaining a detailed history and physical examination. The history and physical examination should attend especially to arterial disease, diabetes, and neuropathies involving sensation. An examination of the genitals should be carried out early by an experienced clinician, preferably of the same sex as the patient, to exclude local pathology such as genital warts, phimosis, vaginismus, testicular pathology. A detailed drug history (prescribed and illicit including alcohol) along with an assessment of personality and relationship history should be obtained. Disorders of sudden onset at the time of a stressor are generally considered psychological. Insidious development of dysfunction indicates a potential organic process especially if there are abnormal findings in the physical examination.

Management for most disorders includes intervening in the psychosomatic cycle of performance anxiety and poor performance. A Masters and Johnson approach is the most common one advocated and includes a behavioural approach with clear homework tasks based on mutually agreed goals. This involves an initial ban on sex to break the psychosomatic cycle. Graded exposure is a technique whereby each partner learns to rediscover what actually arouses them starting with just non-genital touch and massage. This needs to be carefully planned during homework sessions to ensure that there are no interruptions; both partners make sure they are available and must see the session times as protected time into which no other business intrudes. Spending this time together on non-sexual matters also aids communication. Gradually focused genital sensation is reached by mutual agreement. The usual difficulty is to ensure that the pace is kept slow so that a couple do not 'miss out the non-genital' components. Help with negotiation and communication further helps each of the partners to frankly discuss how they are feeling and which behaviours they wish were different.[2] For further reading see ref. 3.

Erectile failure (see ref. 4)

This is defined as persistent failure to sustain an erection of sufficient rigidity for penetrative intercourse. The prevalence is associated with age and affects up to one-third of the over 65s. Erectile failure is the common outcome of several possible causal factors: psychological, neurological, vascular, endocrinological (including hormonal), traumatic, prescribed and other drug use (excessive alcohol consumption).

Peripheral nerve lesions (especially of sacral outflow S2–4) including cauda equina lesions along with CNS pathology (multiple sclerosis or spinal cord lesion) can cause erectile failure. Testosterone levels are rarely too low but there is an age-associated decline. Low testosterone usually affects the sex drive but is not solely responsible for erectile failure. High prolactin also affects libido and can arise with prescribed medications (always consider this and consult the *British National Formulary*) or physiologically alongside a low testosterone. Those who have arterial disease or risk factors (diabetes, hypertension, smoking, family history of heart disease and risk factors, high lipid levels) are especially likely to develop erectile failure of vascular origin. Psychologically caused erectile failure usually arises suddenly with normal ejaculation and continuing early morning erections. Erectile failure may also abate with another partner or during masturbation. Organic causes usually take effect slowly and, classically, early morning erections are absent.

The drugs associated with erectile failure include:

- Antihypertensives
- Antidepressants
- Antipsychotics
- Lithium
- Steroids
- Oestrogens
- Cimetidine

Treatments are directed at the cause but it is likely that there will always be a psychological component. Better diabetic management and alterations of antihypertensives requires effective liaison with the endocrine, medical, neurology and urology specialists. Blood chemistry including glucose, urea and electrolytes and thyroid function should be investigated. Papaverine intracavernosally is often used as a diagnostic test to exclude a vascular cause. Furthermore in some instances this can be continued as a treatment but may produce fibrosis when administered chronically and there is a risk of priapism. Patients need to be trained to self-administer safely and only those experienced in its use should offer it as a treatment if all other interventions fail. Intracavernosal papaverine may also demonstrate impalpable Peyronie's disease as might Doppler imaging. Urology assessment will involve ultrasonography which can identify potentially repairable (surgically) venous leaks. There are also vacuum devices and surgical implants, which may be wanted by some groups (e.g. young men with spinal cord injury).

Premature ejaculation

This is defined as ejaculation that seems involuntary and occurs before both partners are sexually satisfied. There is no magic time against which 'premature' is measured and this disorder may be better defined as a mismatch between partners during sexual activity. Performance anxiety after a single episode may compound and hence perpetuate the problem. Premature ejaculation of course is common amongst the young and sexually inexperienced. Premature ejaculation is not a sign of organic illness. It must be distinguished from retarded or absent ejaculation, which can arise in diabetes, neurological disorders (multiple sclerosis, spinal cord lesions, neuropathies), after prostatectomy and due to prescribed medications. Again neuroleptics, especially thioridazine, are implicated. Indeed thioridazine has been used to treat premature ejaculation in small doses. More recently the SSRIs, despite being implicated in some sexual dysfunctions (orgasmic dysfunction), have also been used to treat sexual disorders caused by anxiety.

Anorgasmia

This is defined as persistent failure of orgasm despite normal arousal. The time required for women to become sufficiently aroused varies and is usually longer than in men. Partner arousal time mismatch may be responsible. Some require manual clitoral stimulation before intercourse. The ability to reach an orgasm manually or with other partners makes it more likely that there is an arousal time mismatch rather than orgasmic failure. Anorgasmia is especially common in young women. An assessment includes physical examination for chronic gynaecological disorders such as vaginitis, endometriosis and pelvic inflammatory disease and also for the following:

- General physical illness
- Endocrine: adrenal insufficiency, diabetes, pituitary failure, hypothyroid
- Drugs: antipsychotics and antidepressants
- Spinal cord lesions

Anorgasmia in men needs to be distinguished from retrograde ejaculation and absent ejaculation. This is uncommon in men and is often associated with impaired arousal and/or medications. Otherwise neurological disorders should be excluded.

Vaginismus

This is defined as the painful spasm of the pelvic floor muscles, which prevents penetration. This should be distinguished from vaginal or pelvic infection, or a failure of vaginal lubrication. Usually this arises in young women with no sexual experience at their first attempt at intercourse; even passing the tip of their finger into the vagina results in spasm. This is often repeated at the time of vaginal examination; the treatment is to use increasing grades of dilators from small to large to expose the woman gradually to penetration. The longer the dilator is retained the further the spasm diminishes. This has proved to be effective in the management of vaginismus when other factors have been eliminated. For example, there may be severe relationship difficulties that need to be tackled at the same time or the vaginismus may start after a traumatic event.

Sleep problems

Insomnia

One-third of adults have problems falling asleep. Almost 40% of the elderly have disrupted sleep patterns. Inadequate sleep is associated with a higher mortality although each individual's needs can be shaped. Insomnia can be mild and related to shift-work or acute stress; serious illness or persistent stress leads to longer term sleep disturbance. Those who are chronically poor sleepers may have severe anxiety and depressive disorders, chronic pain or severe physical illness. The problem is essentially one of initiating and maintaining sleep and is operationally defined in DSM-III-R.

Basic treatment involves improving sleep hygiene: avoid stimulants (caffeine), regulate times of sleep and waking, a comfortable environment, avoid other activities in the bedroom (study, TV), avoid alcohol, use relaxation techniques and exercises but avoid strenuous exercise. The active management of pain and reducing physical disability so as to enable patients to take some regular exercise is essential. Avoid napping during the day. Reassure the patient that if they do not sleep, they will not become ill. Usually patients worry about sleeping and this makes it less likely that they sleep. They should plan the sequence of hot drink (caffeine free), relaxation, reading and return to bed should they not sleep. Most importantly they should not lie in the following day or nap during the day.

Hypersomnia

This is defined as excessive sleep associated with somnolence during the day. Narcolepsy is defined as sleep attacks associated with sleep drunkenness on wakening; occupational or social functioning is compromised with catalepsy. Usually begins in adolescence and there is an equal male to female ratio. It is characterized by the patient going from an awake state into REM sleep. Cataplexy, sleep attacks, hypnagogic hallucinations and automatic behaviour are other common features. This is an association with HLA DR2. Differential diagnosis includes primary idiopathic, mental illness (depression, schizophrenia if hallucinating), sleep apnoea and organic factors (e.g. hypothyroidism). Investigations in sleep laboratories establish the REM latency and video recordings help with the differential diagnosis of other sleep disorders (see below: nightmares, sleep walking). Methylphenidate or tranylcypromine have been successfully used to manage narcolepsy. Accompanying cataplexy is treated with a small dose of antidepressant.

Nightmares

These are characterized by emotional and physiological arousal but with loss of muscular tone (paralysis) characteristic of REM sleep. The subject will remember being unable to move as he/she wakes. The dream is vivid and remembered on wakening. The dreamer may be a little confused on wakening.

Night terrors

These occur in slow wave sleep (usually stage 4) and hence start within a couple of hours of sleep onset. They are unusual in adulthood but can occur at times of stress. Children usually grow out of them.

Partial arousal from sleep is accompanied by intense fear associated with psychological responses to fear: tachycardia, hyperventilation, perspiration. They can be precipitated by external noise or internal states. These same states may repeatedly trigger the episodes in one individual. Head injury, systemic illness (especially febrile states), drug and alcohol intoxication may be of importance in their onset in some individuals. There may be a series of screams or groans and physical movement may be that of escape activity, although usually the person simply sits in bed. Occasionally violent acts can be carried out but this is unusual.

Sleepwalking

Usually starts in childhood and adults suffering from it usually do so, as in the case of night terrors, at times of stress, drug and alcohol intoxication and after head injury. It usually occurs in stages 3 and 4 and hence within the first few hours of sleep onset. There may be small repetitive movements of the sleepwalker, who can wander around the bedroom or even outside by negotiating barriers like doors, etc. There is then invariably a danger that the sleepwalker may injure themselves, walk into traffic, climb out of a window, etc. Contrary to popular opinion sleepwalkers can carry out purposeful and complex acts that are responsive to their environment and only after careful observation may a patient's partner conclude that they are in fact asleep. There is often a family history. Management involves avoiding stressors, knowing triggers for that individual (alcohol for example), sleep hygiene and avoiding medication if possible. Benzodiazepines may exacerbate sleep apnoea, and can produce hangover effects, dependency and rebound anxiety.

REFERENCES

1   Read, S. G. (ed.) (in press) *Psychiatry in Learning Difficulties.* W. B. Saunders.

2   Crowe, M. & Ridley, J. (1990) *Therapy with Couples. A Behavioural Systems Approach.* Oxford: Blackwell Scientific.

3   Bancroft, J. (1983) *Human Sexuality and its Problems.* Edinburgh: Churchill Livingstone.

4   Kirby (1994) Impotence: diagnosis and management of male erectile dysfunction. *British Medical Journal* **308**, 957–960.

Section IX
Therapeutics

PHYSICAL TREATMENTS

Drug treatments

In this section a basic outline of clinical pharmacology is presented with an introduction about drug absorption, metabolism and excretion. For a more detailed discussion of individual drugs readers are referred to the latest edition of the *British National Formulary*.

Pharmacokinetics

Pharmacokinetics is defined as the study of the absorption, distribution, metabolism and excretion of drugs and the time course of these processes. An understanding of these processes encourages rational prescribing.[1] Physical illness can also affect each of these processes.[2]

Absorption

Bioavailability. This is the relative amount of administered drug reaching the systemic circulation and the rate at which this occurs.

Factors influencing bioavailability

- Drug characteristics (e.g. instability, ionization)
- Formulation characteristics (e.g. compression and physical factors affect dissolution)
- Interactions (e.g. food or drugs in gut)
- Patient characteristics (e.g. gut disease – malabsorption, gut motility)

Sustained-release preparations. The advantages include: prolonged effects, improved compliance, comparable or improved efficacy, improved tolerability. Such preparations are of special value if drug has a short half-life, prolonged treatment is necessary or constant plasma levels are needed.

The disadvantages include: cost, delayed absorption so slower onset of effect, prolonged toxicity, risk of overdose, increased toxicity at site of absorption (e.g. gut, skin, muscle).

Routes of drug administration

1. Sublingual
2. Rectal
3. Intramuscular:
   (a) avoids first-pass metabolism
   (b) absorption influenced by local blood flow
   (c) physical properties of the drug (e.g. phenytoin precipitates in muscle)
   (d) sex of patient
   (e) site
   (f) compliance ensured
   (g) onset of action more rapid than oral route
   (h) prolonged absorption with sustained-release preparations
   (i) complications: skin necrosis, abscess, sciatic nerve damage, pain, inadvertent intravenous injection, elevated CPK
4. Intravenous:
   (a) bioavailability immaterial
   (b) instantaneous response
   (c) rate of administration flexible
   (d) drug cannot be recalled
   (e) only water-soluble drugs or aqueous mixtures can be given
   (f) local irritant properties of drug important

(g) risks of anaphylaxis, infection, tissue damage

Most antidepressants and neuroleptics are lipid soluble, poorly ionized in the gut and absorbed by passive diffusion, whereas lithium is ionized and absorbed by an active carrier system. Drug interactions with concomitant medications can slow absorption from the gut (anticholinergic activity; antacids/food in stomach) or speed it up (thyrotoxicosis, gastroenteritis). Diazepam is poorly absorbed by intramuscular route and lorazepam is the preferred drug for rapid intramuscular sedation.

Distribution and protein binding

Volume of distribution. This is a theoretical concept which assumes that the body is a single compartment with the drug evenly distributed throughout it and equals the amount of drug in the body divided by the plasma drug concentration. For highly protein-bound or fat-soluble drugs this figure is large.

Highly protein-bound drugs are more susceptible to changes in binding state. In low-protein states oral dose needs to be decreased. Protein-bound drug might be displaced (anticonvulsants, antidepressants and neuroleptics). Lithium is not protein bound and has a volume of distribution just larger than total body water. Anything affecting fluid balance therefore will influence plasma lithium concentrations (diarrhoea, diuretics).

Metabolism

Phase 1: modification (oxidation, reduction, hydrolysis).
Phase 2: conjugation (with glucuronic acid, glycine, glutamine, sulphate, acetate).

Metabolic derivatives may be more or less active than parent compound, with different half-lives: e.g. amitriptyline is converted to nortriptyline, imipramine is converted to desipramine.

First-pass metabolism in liver or gut wall is especially important if drug is lipid bound. Thus only 30% of an oral dose of chlorpromazine is absorbed because the rest is metabolized in the liver on first pass. Hence if a lipid-bound drug is given parenterally the dose needs to be reduced accordingly.

Pharmacogenetics. Slow and fast metabolism of some drugs (e.g. phenelzine) is influenced by acetylator status, which is genetically determined. Rapid acetylation has autosomal dominant inheritance. Its prevalence varies across ethnic groups (18% in Egyptians to 100% in Canadian Eskimos). Cytochrome P450 shows variation between individuals and one of these enzyme systems is especially influential in psychotropic metabolism. People with the *CYP2D2* allele variant (up to 10% of the population) show high blood levels of psychotropic drug and are therefore more likely to have adverse effects. The elderly have a slower rate of metabolism, and are more sensitive to the effects of a drug (pharmacodynamic effect).

Hepatic function. Liver disease impairs the breakdown of drugs and prolongs the effects of active drug. Enzyme induction speeds up and enzyme inhibition slows down drug metabolism (barbiturates or phenytoin enhance metabolism of antidepressants while neuroleptics such as chlorpromazine inhibit the metabolism of antidepressants).

Excretion

Half-life. This is defined as the time taken for the blood concentration to diminish by 50%. Most drugs are eliminated by 'first-order kinetics': the amount of drug eliminated is proportional to the amount of drug there is in the body. It takes about five half-lives to reach steady state. The frequency of daily administration also is dependent on the half-life: drugs with a short half-life need to be given more frequently. Clinically effective dosage schedules can therefore be worked out.

Clearance. This is the volume of biological fluid cleared of drug per unit time, i.e. rate of elimination/plasma concentration. Age and renal disease can affect clearance.

Renal excretion. Most drugs are eliminated by the kidneys as inactive metabolites after they have been conjugated. Lithium is excreted without any metabolic changes. Over 60% of lithium in the filtrate is reabsorbed in the proximal convoluted tubule and competes with sodium. Sodium depletion therefore can lead to lithium toxicity.

Neuroleptics

This class of drugs has been available since the 1950s and is mainly used to treat schizophrenia, organic psychoses and mania.

Class	Subgroup based on structure	Example drug
Phenothiazines	Aliphatic side-chain	Chlorpromazine, promazine
	Piperidine side-chain	Thioridazine
	Piperazine side-chain	Trifluoperazine, prochlorperazine
Thioxanthenes		Flupenthixol, zuclopenthixol
Butyrophenones		Haloperidol, droperidol
Diphenylbutylpiperidine		Pimozide
Substituted benzamides		Sulpiride
Dibenzoxazepine		Loxapine

Antipsychotics: equivalent dose and adverse effect (from ref. 3)

Drug	Equivalent (mg)	Sedation	Extrapyramidal side-effects	Anticholinergic	Cardiovascular
Chlorpromazine	100	+++	++	++	+++
Promazine	200	+++	+	++	++
Thioridazine	100	+++	+	+++	+++
Fluphenazine	2	+	+++	++	+
Perphenazine	10	+	+++	+	+
Trifluoperazine	5	+	+++	+/−	+
Flupenthixol	3	+	++	++	+
Zuclopenthixol	25	++	++	++	+
Haloperidol	3	+	+++	+	+
Droperidol	4	++	+++	+	+
Benperidol	0.25	+	+++	+	+
Sulpiride	200	−	+	+	−
Pimozide	2	+	+	+	+++
Loxapine	10	++	+++	+	++
Clozapine	50	+++	−	+++	+++
Risperidone	2	+	?	+	+

Depot: adverse effects as for oral preparations

Fluphenazine	5/week
Pipothiazine	10/week
Haloperidol	15/week
Flupenthixol	10/week
Zuclopenthixol	100/week

Mechanism

Antipsychotic activity is directly proportional to dopamine blockade but also to blockade to varying degrees of adrenergic, cholinergic, serotonergic and histamine receptors. Sites of dopamine blockade (and effects) include: striatum (extrapyramidal symptoms and motor effects), limbic forebrain and neocortex (antipsychotic activity), hypothalamus (raised prolactin levels) and brainstem (antiemetic action on chemoreceptor trigger zone).

Adverse effects

Sedation: ataractic state, depression, confusion

Increased appetite and weight gain

Motor manifestations: parkinsonian extrapyramidal symptoms, acute dystonias, akathisia, chronic administration can lead to tardive dyskinesias

Neuroleptic malignant syndrome: occurs in 0.5% of newly treated patients; 20% mortality. Symptoms include hyperthermia, muscular rigidity, labile blood pressure, raised white count, raised CPK

Anti-adrenergic effects: alpha-1-receptor blockade leads to hypotension and tachycardia, blurred vision, delayed or inhibited ejaculation, nasal stuffiness

Hypothalamic effects: hyperprolactinaemia, impotence, galactorrhoea, gynaecomastia, hypothermia, heat stroke

Anticholinergic effects: diplopia, dry mouth, urinary retention, constipation, cardiac conduction block or delay, arrhythmias

Lower seizure threshold leading to epileptic fits

Allergic reactions: cholestatic jaundice, urticaria, dermatitis, blood dyscrasias, light-sensitive rash

Rare: pigmentary retinopathy (especially thioridazine), corneal and lens opacities, raised cholesterol, diabetes, cardiac arrhythmias, cardiac arrest

Management of adverse effects

Generally choose a drug with the best side-effect profile that the individual patient can tolerate but also to capitalize on the drug effects (e.g sedation may be desirable).

Motor symptoms such as parkinsonian symptoms: use anticholinergics such as procyclidine or benzhexol. Acute dystonias: acute i.m. or slow i.v. procyclidine (5–10 mg). Akathisia: reduce neuroleptic dose; propranolol (20–40 mg two to three times daily) may also be helpful; if severe use a short course of diazepam (5 mg t.d.s.) as a muscle relaxant for symptomatic treatment.

Skin care: avoid sunlight, use plenty of emollients, treat skin rashes early, antihistamines may help.

Neuroleptic malignant syndrome: stop all drugs, seek medical assessment, transfer to ITU if severely ill and dehydrated. Combined administration of the muscle relaxant dantrolene and dopamine agonist bromocriptine reduces mortality and speeds up recovery in some cases but these drugs themselves carry considerable adverse effects.

Atypical antipsychotics

Clozapine

Clozapine belongs to the dibenzoxazepine class of drugs (as does loxapine). It blocks D_2 receptors to a lesser extent than do conventional antipsychotics but also blocks 5-HT_{2a}, 5-HT_{2c}, D_4

and histamine receptors. This profile of receptor occupancy is thought to be the reason for such a low incidence of extrapyramidal side-effects and for its effects on negative symptoms. Between one-third and two-thirds of those resistant to conventional antipsychotics will respond to clozapine over a period of 2 years. The major drawback is the small risk of agranulocytosis, which can be fatal. In the UK for 6316 patients treated with clozapine for up to 48 months, 4% developed a neutropenia and 0.8% agranulocytosis. The risk is greatest in the first 18 weeks of treatment with a further decrease in the frequency of both phenomena after 1 year. To prescribe in the UK a patient must be registered with the clozapine patient monitoring services (CPMS) and have blood taken before commencement of treatment and then weekly for the first 18 weeks, 2-weekly thereafter for 1 year and then 4-weekly if there have been no concerns about low neutrophil counts. Starting doses are usually: day 1, 12.5 mg nocte; day 2, 12.5 mg b.d.; increasing in 12.5 mg increments daily. The CPMS alerts the clinician to a green, amber (or flashing amber) and red alert results: these mean satisfactory, more samples are required, and withdraw the drug, respectively. If the drug is withdrawn, samples must be taken for a further 4 weeks to ensure recovery. If there is a partial response then concomitant haloperidol, sulpiride or risperidone is safe for a trial. Additional neuroleptics especially depot preparations should be avoided if possible. The maximum dose is 900 mg/daily.

Side-effects include hypersalivation, for which an anticholinergic such as hyoscine can be given, hypotension and tachycardia, weight gain, delirium, myocarditis, sedation, nocturnal enuresis and grand mal seizures. In the instance of fits and proven antipsychotic effectiveness prescribe sodium valproate. In view of the risks, for those on a Mental Health Act section involve the family or next of kin in treatment decisions. Taking blood is not clearly covered under the Mental Health Act but as it is necessary to ensure the 'safe' treatment of a patient on clozapine, treatment under the Act is usually interpreted to include taking blood. Not a single test case has yet come to court but the assumption is that blood samples are a necessary part of the treatment.

Risperidone

Risperidone is a strong blocker of 5-HT$_2$ receptors and a weaker blocker of D$_2$ receptors, alpha-1 and alpha-2 adrenergic and H$_1$ histamine receptors. Placebo-controlled trials find it to be as effective as neuroleptics for the treatment of positive and negative symptoms. Dose-response studies indicate a maximal response between 4 and 8 mg a day usually given as a b.d. regimen. Risperidone has fewer extrapyramidal effects than neuroleptics but not less than those of clozapine, although it is less sedating. The half-life is 24 hours (prolonged in the elderly).

Side effects include: extrapyramidal side-effects, weight gain, tachycardia, sexual dysfunction and rebound anxiety or relapse when switching from the more sedative agents too quickly. Also, fatigue, anxiety, nausea, low white count, epilepsy and hyperprolactinaemia.

Benzodiazepines

Mechanism

These drugs are used as anxiolytics, hypnotics, muscle relaxants, anticonvulsants, for myoclonus and for sedation during short operative procedures.

Their powerful anxiolytic action is thought to be mediated by potentiating the action of the inhibitory neurotransmitter GABA. Flumazenil also binds to the same molecular complex and reverses the action of benzodiazepines although its half-life is shorter than many of the benzodiazepines.

	Half-life (hours)	Half-life of metabolite (hours)	Approximate equivalent dose (mg)
Diazepam	20–50	40–200	10
Chlordiazepoxide	5–30	130	20
Lorazepam	10–20	Nil	2
Nitrazepam	28	Nil	20
Temazepam	8	12	20

Benzodiazepines should not be prescribed long term, and only for specific disorders where they are of proven benefit. They are helpful as an adjunct in the treatment of acute psychoses, and severe panic attacks. Where they are used for neurosis a behavioural programme should be initiated and the short-term nature of the pharmacological approach, mainly for crisis intervention, must be clearly established with the patient. For example in the instance of persistent insomnia, sleep hygiene with a reduction of stimulants and intoxicants should be explored. Strict times to awake and go to bed along with relaxation practice are preferred. For persistent anxiety states a low dose of a longer acting preparation is preferable but again prescription should not continue for more than 4 weeks.

Adverse effects

Sedation, fatigue, ataxia, diplopia, dysarthria, inco-ordination, apathy, impaired memory, poor concentration, prolonged reaction times, paradoxical excitement and rage reactions, pseudohallucinations. Anterograde amnesia, falls in the elderly, hangover effects, REM sleep suppression with rebound the following day

Dependence, both psychological and physical. Post-withdrawal states can last many weeks or months. Cases have been reported whereby dependence arose after single dose exposure. There is little cardiovascular or respiratory depression although with alcohol or other CNS depressants this effect is potentiated

Rarely transient hypotension and apnoea

Allergy is uncommon but thrombophlebitis after intravenous administration is accompanied by pain. Intra-arterial administration leads to spasm, ischaemia and possibly gangrene

Alcohol and cimetidine block benzodiazepine metabolism and hepatic or renal failure can contribute to the development of toxicity

Management of withdrawal
The elderly with multiple physical health problems are especially at risk of becoming the new long-term users of benzodiazepines. The Mental Health Foundation guidelines[4] advocate a two-pronged approach: encouraging and managing withdrawal and preventing new cases. Although there are good reasons for continuing prescriptions for patients who are long-term users of benzodiazepines, doctors may overestimate the problems. Continuous treatment cards and prescription monitoring have been advocated as effective interventions. The more potent and shorter acting benzodiazepines carry a greater risk of dependence.

In withdrawal states the following symptoms can occur: irritability, severe anxiety, panic, headache, insomnia, depression, chronic muscle and joint pains, hypersensitivity to light and sound, fits, depersonalization and derealization symptoms, visual and auditory hallucinations, change in smell and taste, tinnitus, flu-like symptoms, formication and frank psychoses. These symptoms can begin within 24 hours if a short-acting benzodiazepine is being used, or up to 2 months if a longer acting one is responsible.

Prevention: avoid high doses for longer than 1–2 months; identify those with a history of previous drug or alcohol addiction or abnormal pre-morbid personalities. Although one should avoid the use of short-acting compounds (alprazolam, lorazepam and triazolam) they are of value in emergencies.

Change to longer acting preparations before withdrawal. If there is a history of fits use an anticonvulsant in the early stages; if fits have occurred during previous withdrawals hospital admission should be considered for the early stages. Cognitive behavioural treatments should be considered. Symptomatic treatment with a beta-blocker and antidepressant may be helpful but do not always allay the withdrawal symptoms. There is no agreed decrement that is suitable for all patients although 0.5–2.5 mg of diazepam has been suggested as most suitable. It is best to titrate symptoms against the amount by which the benzodiazepine is reduced. Withdrawal may take up to 16 weeks in uncomplicated cases but in some symptoms may persist for many years.

Antidepressants

Tricyclics
These are used in major depression, schizoaffective states, phobic anxiety states and other neuroses, enuresis, atypical facial pain and chronic pain.

Mechanism. Tricyclics act by blocking amine (noradrenaline, 5-HT, dopamine) reuptake by presynaptic neurones after neuronal discharge. The clinical effect takes at least 10 days to become manifest, even though in animal studies the blockade of uptake is immediate. The post-synaptic receptor down-regulation in response to higher neurotransmitter concentrations in the synaptic cleft seems to have the same time course as the clinical effect. Tertiary amines undergo hepatic metabolism to produce secondary amine metabolites, which also are active antidepressants.

Drug	Half-life (hours)	Metabolites (half-life in hours)	Other effects
Amitriptyline	8–20	Nortriptyline (20–90)	Sedative, strongly anticholinergic, postural hypotension, tachycardia, arrhythmias especially cardiac if conduction delay; avoid in prostatism, after myocardial infarction, glaucoma
Dothiepin	45–55	None	Fewer anticholinergic and significant anxiolytic effect
Clomipramine	17–28	Desmethyl metabolite	Powerful inhibition of 5-HT uptake; especially useful in phobias
Imipramine	4–8	Desipramine (12–25)	Little sedation, powerful anticholinergic; useful in panic disorder
Lofepramine	1.5–6	Desipramine	Safer in overdose, avoid in pregnancy and lactation; less sedative and cardiotoxic than amitriptyline. Raised liver function tests
Trimipramine	7–23	Desmethyl metabolite	More sedative than amitriptyline. Avoid in young children and pregnancy

Other adverse effects

Tremor, sedation, seizures, hangover effect, headache, myoclonus, paraesthesiae, movement disorders, nightmares, hypomania, acute confusion

Increased appetite, weight gain, paralytic ileus, gastric reflux and acute urinary retention

Anticholinergic effects: blurred vision, dry mouth, bad taste, constipation, hesitancy, urinary retention, impotence, delayed orgasm, aggravated glaucoma

Cardiac effects: alpha blockade causes hypotension, sexual dysfunction. Palpitations, supraventricular tachyarrhythmias, AV block, bundle branch blocks, T wave and ST depression, prolonged PR, QRS and QT intervals on ECG

Rare: cholestatic jaundice, vasculitis, dermatitis

Monoamine oxidase inhibitors (MAOIs)

These drugs inhibit the action of monoamine oxidases, which usually deactivate neurotransmitters in the nerve terminals after reuptake. They take several weeks to become active when all the stores of MAO are depleted. They are used for atypical depressions and where other antidepressants have failed and are especially useful where anxiety symptoms predominate. MAOI type A inhibit the breakdown of 5-HT and noradrenaline. MAOI type B prevent dopamine breakdown (e.g. selegeline, which is used in parkinsonism).

MAOI	Type	Adverse effects
Phenelzine (hydrazine derivative)	Inactivated by acetylation	Leucopenia, anxiety, agitation, confusion, weight gain, psychosis, hepatotoxicity. Food: avoid tyramine and other sympathomimetics. Avoid: opiates, antidepressants (especially 5-HT blockers). Avoid use in cardiovascular, diabetic and endocrine disorders
Tranylcypromine (non-hydrazine)	Amphetamine-like	More severe food and drug reactions, liver disease less frequently, CNS stimulant/dependency potential common
Moclobemide	Reversible MAO-A inhibitor	Fewer adverse effects and drug interactions. If high doses used then food interactions possible. Avoid: SSRIs, clomipramine, L-dopa, pethidine

Practice points

> Some foods to avoid: cheeses, meats, some wine (Chianti), yeast extracts, some beers (Worthington and Bass), broad bean pods, banana skin, roe, green figs, hung game, Oxo, Marmite, pickled herring, pâté and chicken liver. The combination of a tricyclic antidepressant and an MAOI are only to be used in expert hands for treatment-resistant depression. Avoid clomipramine and tranylcypromine mixtures; avoid antidepressants, which are powerful 5-HT reuptake blockers. It is better to start the tricyclic first in low dose and then add the MAOI. Moclobemide is advocated by the manufacturers as a potential first-line treatment in any depressive state in view of the better safety profile.
>
> Signs of 'cheese reaction': flushing, pounding headache, tachycardia, hypertension. If severe can cause agitation, hallucinations, convulsions, pyrexia, cerebrovascular accident and hyperreflexia. If severe, an alpha-blocker (phentolamine 2-4 mg i.v.) may be necessary. Some advocate the use of chlorpromazine orally or intravenously to reduce the blood pressure but this may lead to cardiovascular complications such as arrhythmias and subsequent severe hypotension.

Selective serotonin reuptake inhibitors
These drugs inhibit the uptake of 5-HT into brain synaptosomes but have very little effect on dopamine and noradrenaline. As such they have fewer side-effects than tricyclics and are much safer in overdose. They are especially helpful in patients with OCD or phobic anxiety states. This group of drugs is better tolerated by elderly patients and the rationale for recommending them as first-line agents is that patients are likely

to better comply with treatment where the adverse effect profile is less aversive than traditional agents.

	Half-life	Half-life of metabolite	Characteristic effects
Fluvoxamine	15 hours	?	Nausea, convulsions, not sedative, akathisia; increased warfarin, theophylline, tricyclic and phenytoin levels
Fluoxetine	1–3 days	7–15 days	Weight loss, rash, anxiety, insomnia, sexual dysfunction, akathisia, impulsive behaviour, safest in epilepsy
Sertraline	25 hours	Nil	No metabolic interactions
Paroxetine	20 hours	66 hours	Useful for refractory depression, slightly sedative, tardive dyskinesia on withdrawal
Citalopram	1.5 days	None significant	The most 5-HT-specific SSRI. Gastrointestinal side-effects as other SSRIs. The most common side-effect is mania

Other adverse effects

Minimal affinity for muscarinic and adrenergic receptors but occasionally anticholinergic and anti-adrenergic effects arise

5-HT effects of bloating, nausea, diarrhoea

Serotonergic syndrome of hyperactivity, agitation, hyperthermia, tachycardia, especially if combined with MAOIs, L-tryptophan and lithium

Lithium Lithium salts are used in the treatment of acute mania (but can take 2 weeks for a response), prophylaxis of bipolar affective disorder, unipolar depressive states, refractory depressive states, self-mutilation in those with learning difficulties, and as an anti-impulse agent in those with any of the impulse disorders. It reduces the number and severity of relapses in bipolar disorders and may help prevent antidepressant-induced hypomania. It is also of value in the treatment of recurrent unipolar depression and in acute depression. However most clinicians prefer to use antidepressants as prophylaxis and as first-line agents in depression, reserving the use of lithium for severely ill patients.

Mechanism
This remains elusive and was thought to involve Na^+/K^+ channel opening and rates of opening in neuronal membranes. Regulation of phosphatidylinositol messenger systems is thought to play an important part. Lithium is not metabolized and is renally excreted.

Practice notes

Therapeutic level monitoring is essential as irreversible renal toxicity can occur above levels of 1.5 mmol l^{-1}. Advised levels for mania: 1.0–1.2 mmol l^{-1}; for prophylaxis 0.6–1.0 mmol l^{-1}. For elderly patients, sodium-depleted patients or those with impaired renal function or CNS disease, or in order to augment antidepressants, lower levels (0.4–0.6 mmol l^{-1}) may suffice

Obtain urea and electrolytes, thyroid function and ECG before commencing treatment. Take levels 12 hours after dose (at a trough). Half-life is 20 hours, which is prolonged in elderly (<36 hours) and with chronic treatment (up to 50 hours)

If toxicity develops, stop lithium, give i.v. saline and osmotic diuresis

Adverse effects

Dose-dependent effects: mild tremor to ataxia, drowsiness, weakness, thirst, diarrhoea to severe tremor, ataxia, dysarthria, nystagmus, spasticity, hyperreflexia, vomiting, confusion, coma, dehydration, death (if >4 mmol l^{-1})

Dose-independent effects: effects on renal and thyroid adenylate cyclase systems causing 4% to develop hypothyroidism (rarely hyperthyroid states have been reported), nephrogenic diabetes insipidus. Thirst, polyuria and hyperaldosteronism. Cardiac conduction delays (ensure no bundle branch block, severe ischaemic heart disease, sick sinus syndrome), may cause arrhythmias. Leucopenia and weight gain also reported. Skin conditions such as psoriasis can be exacerbated during lithium treatment

Secreted in breast milk (contraindicated); if given in first trimester can cause Ebstein's congenital anomaly (low-set tricuspid valve)

Possible toxicity with loop and, in particular, thiazide diuretics, extrapyramidal symptoms commoner with co-prescription of neuroleptic as is likelihood of neuroleptic malignant syndrome with high-dose haloperidol. Co-prescription of nonsteroidal anti-inflammatory drugs, phenylbutazone and tetracyclines can impair renal secretion

Carbamazepine

Carbamazepine originally was used as an anticonvulsant for grand mal and focal seizures. It is also used in trigeminal neuralgia, phantom limb pain, alcohol withdrawal and episodic dyscontrol syndrome as well as for irritability in any psychiatric condition. Anticonvulsants have a truly antimanic effect and are used when lithium and/or neuroleptics have been unsuccessful.

Sodium valproate also has anticonvulsant and antimanic properties. It is most effective in rapid cycling patients who usually do not respond to lithium treatment. Combination therapy may be necessary in such patients.

Practice notes

Its clinical effects can take 2 weeks to develop; it can be used alone or in combination with lithium. Serum levels of 8–12 mmol l⁻¹ are optimal although some patients will respond at lower levels. Carbamazepine is an enzyme inducer. Its half-life is 30 hours but on chronic dosing is 12 hours. It has weak antidepressant properties and in view of a similar structure to tricyclic antidepressants, ensure a washout period before administration after an MAOI.

Adverse effects

Drowsiness, ataxia, diplopia, dysarthria

Aplastic anaemia (1 in 20 000), agranulocytosis (warn patients about fever and obtain pretreatment and regular full blood counts)

Hypersensitivity, rashes (3%), inappropriate antidiuretic hormone syndrome leading to hyponatraemia

Raised alkaline phosphatase and gamma-glutamyl transferase indicate hypersensitivity so stop treatment as this can become generalized hypersensitivity leading to hepatitis

Avoid in pregnancy and breast-feeding

As carbamazepine is an enzyme inducer it can render oral contraceptive and other anticonvulsants ineffective (can also cause anticonvulsant toxicity)

Raised drug levels of cimetidine, calcium channel

blockers, erythromycin, fluoxetine and dextro-propoxyphene

Neurotoxic reactions, although uncommon, can occur when used with lithium

Electroconvulsive therapy

Indications for ECT treatment include major depression with psychosis, major depression where a quick response is essential (severe weight loss or stupor), puerperal psychoses, catatonic schizophrenia, major depression not responding to drug treatment, where it is uncertain whether the symptoms presented are consistent with a depressive state (especially in the elderly and in medical conditions where oral medication is not tolerated) and finally in acute mania that does not respond to other interventions.

Mechanism

Both the waveform and energy used influence the outcome. Biphasic sine waves and uniphasic constant current are the most effective. High-energy pulses are more effective than low-energy pulses. For the optimal therapeutic effect the electrical seizure must be bilateral (the exact duration required is disputed). Although not common in this country EEG monitoring is advocated by some and is routine practice in some states in North America. A sphygmo-manometer cuff to prevent the passage of muscle relaxant into the forearm may be used to examine visually the onset and termination of a seizure and hence the duration, which should be at least 20–25 seconds. There is an increase in cerebral blood flow by up to 200%. An initial bradycardia is followed by a sudden tachycardia; the heart rate then falls to just below resting and then there is sustained slight tachycardia for minutes. With muscle relaxants the blood pressure does not rise to extremes but the systolic can still occasionally reach 200 mmHg.

The exact therapeutic component remains elusive. During the procedure neurochemical changes include elevated levels of tryptophan, raised MAO activity and increased blood–brain barrier permeability. Prolactin is raised 20 minutes after a seizure; this rise attenuates as treatment proceeds but is sometimes measured to ensure a seizure took place. Elevation of oxytocin-related neurophysin after ECT has been demonstrated in at least one study to correlate with improvement. There is increased cortisol and ACTH release but growth hormone and thyroid stimulating hormone are not usually affected. The EEG shows a build-up of diffuse, irregular, low-frequency activity, with delta and some theta activity. There is greater REM sleep, reduced REM latency and a reduction in total sleep time.

Receptor	ECT	Antidepressants
5-HT$_1$	Decreased	Decreased
5-HT$_2$	Increased	Decreased
Dopamine	No change	
GABA	Increased	Increased
Beta adrenergic	Decreased	Decreased
Alpha-2 adrenergic	Decreased	Decreased
Alpha-1 adrenergic	No change	

Practice notes

ECT is contraindicated in raised intracranial pressure, recent intracranial bleed, cerebral/aortic aneurysm, recent myocardial infarction, acute chest infections and in anyone who is unfit for a general anaesthetic. Studies demonstrate that despite a big placebo effect, ECT is effective. The onset of the response is quicker than when drug treatment is used. Bilateral treatment although better produces more post-ECT confusion than unilateral treatment. The latter should only be used if there is severe post-ECT confusion and then is administered to the non-dominant side. Between four and six treatments are usually necessary for a minimal response to be seen. A maximum of 12 treatments is usual. ECT is optimally given on two or three occasions a week; progress should be reviewed weekly and notes made about the seizure type, duration (The Royal College of Psychiatrists advises that a fit of at least 25 seconds duration is efficacious), anaesthetic agents and any complications. If a fit does not visibly occur, check with the anaesthetist that the patient is adequately sedated, and try again at a higher voltage. If this fails do not try for a third time. Note that fit threshold increases as a treatment proceeds. Higher currents may need to be delivered if a fit does not occur or the duration of the fit for any one current setting is falling. ECT machines often do not have adequate control to ensure that a constant current is delivered or that the stimulus is not much greater than required to reach the fit threshold; this minimizes memory impairment.

Urea and electrolytes should be obtained before starting ECT and a thorough physical examination is necessary to exclude the possibility of cardiac and chest disease. Pulse/blood pressure records should be made. An ECG and a chest X-ray should be obtained in the elderly and in those with physical illness. If cerebral disease such as aneurysm or a space-occupying lesion is suspected a CT should be obtained; atypical presentations in which organic brain syndromes are suspected also should have a CT. The patient should be fasted as for any general anaesthetic (at least 6 hours) and should be well hydrated (better fits). All patients (especially day patients) should specifically be asked about the last time they ate. Pre-oxygenation (hyperventilation) by the anaesthetist also facilitates seizure activity. Pre-meds of anticholinergics have traditionally been given but are now less often used. Other medications such as anticonvulsants, benzodiazepines and tryptophan are likely to increase the fit threshold. Handedness should be identified if unilateral placement is considered necessary. In right-handed people the left hemisphere is nearly always dominant whereas in left-handed people the left hemisphere is dominant in 25–50% of cases. Training in electrode placement, types of machine and post-seizure management should be provided before anyone attempts to apply the treatment. In some centres ambulatory ECG monitoring and pulse oximetry are the norm. The college guidelines advise that a separate recovery room should be available and a separate waiting room from that in which treatment takes place. While under anaesthetic a nurse should attend each patient whilst in the recovery position. Success rates of over 70–80% with ECT, 60–70% with antidepressants and 20–30% with placebo have been demonstrated. Relapse rates do not differ. Maintenance treatment with antidepressants is advised as patients may relapse after a successful trial of ECT.

Adverse effects

Confusion (1/4), headache (1/2), amnesia (both retrograde and anterograde recede within 3 months of the treatment), muscle pain, burns, urinary incontinence, broken teeth, vertebral fracture, cardiac arrhythmias, myocardial infarction, cerebral haemorrhage, aspiration pneumonia, pulmonary embolus. The traumatic injuries are far less common now because of the use of muscle relaxants and brief anaesthesia with an anaesthetist present. Lasting memory impairment is unlikely; in those complaining of persistent memory problems it seems these are often due to persistent depressive symptoms.

Psychosurgery

About 20–30 operations are performed annually in two centres in the UK. Most of these are stereotactic subcaudate tractotomies (SSTs, all at the Geoffrey Knight Unit, Brook General Hospital) although some are stereotactic limbic leucotomies (SLLs, mostly at Atkinson Morley). Amygdalotomy is done for pathological aggression; SST for depression, OCD, and occasionally for treatment-resistant anxiety symptoms. SLL is usually done for OCD and disorders involving refractory obsessive symptoms.

Such treatment is only administered if the patient has been exposed to all other possible treatments for the optimal lengths of time and drug doses. Thus for those with depression, each patient is assessed as if they had resistant depression. This involves a reappraisal of the symptoms, history, neurological state and review of the treatments tried and their potential efficacy. If all treatments have not been exhausted then these are attempted prior to operative treatment. Thus a series of pharmacological treatments at high dose and with necessary adjunctive treatments are attempted. For severe depression, this amounts to high-dose clomipramine, with lithium and L-tryptophan on a named-patient basis, possibly adding tri-iodothyronine and an adequate trial of ECT. Severe dementia, personality disorders and severe physical illness that makes the anaesthetic procedure hazardous are contraindications. Assessment is made by a neurosurgeon and a psychiatrist with special knowledge of this field. The procedure has now been considerably refined: radioactive yttrium seeds are located at the targeted site using a stereotactic frame.

Some clinicians argue that there is not a place for such a treatment in modern practice; others argue that it is necessary in severe intractable disorders where other approaches have failed and where there is severe distress and the suicide risk is high.[5] Improvement rates are approximately 70% for depression and 50–60% for anxiety states including OCD. Limbic leucotomy is though to be better for OCD with response rates of over 80%. The absence of control groups (ethical dilemma) makes a rigorous assessment difficult but in view of the refractory nature of the disorders comparison of outcome can be made using cases as their own controls. More work needs to be done on examining the social and psychological outcomes of patients undergoing this treatment. All patients undergoing the procedure must be able to give informed consent. If they cannot (some of the most severely ill) then the Mental Health Act does not allow such treatment to be given. Two independent doctors must agree that the patient is able to give consent.

Adverse effects

Incontinence, apathy, seizures (2%), memory impairment, personality change (very rare), weight gain (very rare), disinhibition, death (1/1200)

PSYCHOLOGICAL TREATMENTS

Psychological treatments are considered essential by most users of psychiatric services. Dissatisfaction has been expressed with purely pharmaceutical treatments offered by both primary and specialist health-care providers, and in recent years there has been a rapid expansion in counsellors employed by GPs, and in forms of psychological treatment being offered that claim to help a wider range of patients and are cheaper and faster than traditional analytically informed psychotherapy. The requirements of the Royal College of Psychiatrists reflect this, stating that trainees must gain experience in a number of different models of psychological intervention. In considering what psychological treatment might be most appropriate for a patient, both the form of treatment and the context (individual, couple, family or group) are important.

Forms of psychological treatment

Forms of psychological treatment tend to lie on a continuum of both length of treatment and depth of work. The divisions shown below are therefore somewhat arbitrary, and overlap occurs. There is no suggestion that one form of treatment is better than another: each patient and set of circumstances needs to be carefully assessed. Indeed, the most complex forms of psychological treatment can be the most inappropriate for many patients – crisis intervention might be totally appropriate for an acutely psychotic patient with schizophrenia, but clearly a formal analysis would not.

Psychoeducation

This form of psychological treatment is appropriate, possibly essential, in any form of mental illness. It is a process that involves two stages. Firstly, a health-care professional, as the expert on psychopathology and treatment, informs the patient, plus his or her carers and support network, about the illness with which he or she has been diagnosed. This will involve full details of likely symptoms, illness patterns, treatment options, preventative measures and prognosis. Secondly, the patient, as the expert on his or her unique experience of the illness, needs to be given time to inform the professionals about his or her symptoms, beliefs about causation, details of what the patient has found likely to improve or worsen symptoms, feelings, fears, and the effect of the illness on his or her daily functioning. This bidirectional flow of information means that a management plan can be negotiated that is individually tailored, acceptable to the patient, and which offers optimal chances of amelioration of, or recovery from, symptoms. The plan will pay particular attention to enabling the patient to recognize warning signs of deterioration or relapses, will encourage strategies for coping with the illness, and for obtaining appropriate support when required. Psychoeducation is particularly important in chronic relapsing mental illnesses such as schizophrenia, where it can be the factor that persuades a reluctant patient to comply with long-term medication, with a proven benefit on number and seriousness of relapses and reduced number of admissions. It is also a process offering immense benefits to families with a psychotic individual, as it enables the family to develop realistic expectations, to support professionals in their advised management plan, and prevents the development of anxiety and high emotional expression, which also contributes to the reduction in expected relapses.

Crisis intervention

Whether a patient suffers from a long-term relapsing mental illness or is generally psychologically stable, a life crisis can intervene leading to anxiety, distress and diminished self-esteem, which can rapidly escalate to symptomatic proportions. A crisis has been described as 'any problem which seems insurmountable and beyond normal coping mechanisms'. Continuing inability to resolve a crisis can lead to exhaustion and progressive deterioration in mental well-being and social functioning. A person can be helped through a crisis by informal or professional support. Research has shown the protective value of a trusted friend or confidante in relapsing depression. All mental health professionals, those who work in casualty departments and general practice staff can be trained in basic techniques of crisis intervention, which may need to be offered on one occasion, or which may need to be formalized into a short course of focused psychological treatment.

Assessment of a person suspected of deteriorating due to a crisis will need to take account of any past history of mental illness, perceived problems, steps already taken to alleviate the situation, and the success or otherwise of these. It will also need to include details of secondary problems, the level of support available to the person in crisis, and details of how the person has coped in the past. Depending on the level of functioning, the client in crisis may only require an empathic ear, support in decision making, and help in planning a stepwise strategy to deal with the crisis. Crisis intervention can be quite directive and advice may be given. If the client is reaching a level of decompensation, where they are not sleeping, their mental state is deteriorating and their functioning in society is severely affected, it may be necessary for a professional or mental health team to temporarily take control and sort out the first steps of a crisis resolution plan for the client. This may enable the client to recuperate sufficiently to begin to engage in the process of forming more successful coping strategies to enable resolution themselves.

Often, crisis intervention requires a high initial input but for a relatively short period. A key-worker may need to network with other agencies and ensure cooperation between them, and often needs to meet with a client's family and support network. Sometimes, it may be necessary to enable a client to move out of a very stressful situation, and a psychiatric admission is not necessarily inappropriate if this would be the most rapid and efficient way of ensuring adequate service input and restoring the client to a better functioning level. Enormous stress can be transferred on to the professional dealing with a case, and team working and support is essential to alleviate this. Specific crisis intervention agencies exist to help with such problems as alcohol or drug relapse, and for victims of violent or sexual incidents. Such agencies hold expert knowledge of both appropriate interventions and available services.

Counselling

Counselling is usually offered by non-medical staff. General principles of counselling are that it is non-directive, non-judgemental, empathic, supportive, and that it enables a client to cope more effectively with their current life circumstances or inner state. Clients find it helpful to air their problems, ventilate their feelings, and feel heard and held. They may gain a new perspective on their difficulties and discover new resources with which they can deal with them. It can be useful as a form of support at times of traumatic life events in the psychologically well, and can also offer help to those with chronic conditions in terms of increasing coping abilities.

Many different models of counselling exist, but counsellors in the UK have generally been accredited through the British Association for Counselling, and therefore subscribe to a code of ethics and practice and have been trained through a recognized organization with a certain number of supervised hours of practice.

Routes to counselling are numerous: many GPs now employ counsellors, counselling training organizations offer low-cost counselling with their trainees, private counsellors advertise and are listed on professional registers, many social workers and nurses have additional counselling qualifications, and specialist counsellors are employed by voluntary organizations, rehabilitation centres, etc.

When a client requests 'talking treatment', he or she is generally referring to counselling. Counselling can be at many different levels. A short course of supportive sessions could be appropriate for almost anyone, from a usually well but recently bereaved professional person, to a carer of someone with a major disability, to someone with a long-term mental illness experiencing particular worries. Supportive counselling aims to offer reassurance, facilitate understanding and to enable a client to function more effectively. It would offer very limited opportunities for cognitive restructuring, unlike insight-oriented therapies such as psychoanalysis.

Counselling can be more insight-oriented and work at deeper levels. In this format, a client would need to show a degree of psychological mindedness, a willingness to look at their own agency in negative situations, and a desire for positive change. Such work, by its nature, tends to be longer. It would not be recommended for borderline or psychotic patients. Counsellors in general practice may only be able to work in a time-limited fashion and potential clients often need to seek private help, or to obtain help from a specialist mental health team.

A referral to a counsellor should consider the counsellor's qualifications and level of supervision, as well as the length of contract they would be willing to offer.

Psychodynamically informed psychotherapy

Though the border between counselling and psychotherapy is blurred, and though both offer support, the essential core of psychotherapy is that it encourages the formation of a meaningful relationship between the client and therapist, which is then used as the context within which psychological defences can be confronted, the past can be recalled and understood, interpersonal dynamics can be explored, regression can take place, unconscious phenomena can be interpreted and conflicts can be acted out and resolved within the therapeutic relationship. Psychotherapy would aim to enable the client to bring about both outer and inner changes.

Psychotherapists do not need to be medically qualified in the UK. As in counselling, many models of theory, practice and training exist; and therapists can practice privately or be employed by the health-care provider. Psychotherapy departments linked to psychiatric departments often offer an assessment service, both to assess the suitability of a referred client for psychotherapy, and to determine which model and mode of delivery would be most appropriate.

Brief focused psychotherapy

This form of psychotherapy is gaining popularity in the UK currently, with research showing positive results in a number of different mental health problems. This treatment appeals to both clients, who understandably seek rapid results, and purchasers of services, who seek efficient, cost-effective, time-limited interventions. The principles behind brief focused therapy are that the therapist works in a psychodynamically informed way, sessions are geared towards insight into current problems and their links with past experiences and personality patterns, and that there is a high level of intervention from the therapist. Homework tasks may be set. To be suitable, clients need to have circumscribed difficulties, a high level of motivation for change, and a capacity for self-reflection. Contracts are often established for six sessions at a time, with an average of 25–30 weekly 1-hour sessions bringing improvement in a number of the neuroses, PTSD, and other disorders.

Insight-oriented/exploratory psychodynamic psychotherapy

Within the therapeutic relationship, the unconscious is explored. Patients are offered regular, time-delineated sessions in a consistent setting. The therapist remains strictly neutral, does not offer advice, and encourages free association. The patient's resistance and defence mechanisms are challenged, confronted, and modified. Transference is fostered, revealed, and interpreted, enabling re-enactment and remembering of early formative experiences. Dreams and fantasies are interpreted. Some models of psychotherapy use specific techniques to access the unconscious such as guided imagery and symbolic representation. Insights gained enable the patient to develop a more whole view of him or herself and his or her relationships with others, so that choices can be made about discarding outmoded ways of thinking and behaving, and developing more optimal ways of functioning.

Suitability for specialist psychotherapy will involve a high level of motivation and commitment, a desire to learn more about oneself, psychological mindedness (sensing links between current difficulties and past traumas, for example), the capacity to enter into a relationship with a therapist and use this fully, an ability to tolerate anxiety, the capacity to be objective and the ability to respond to interpretations. Unsuitability would include psychotic or borderline psychopathology (except when treated by experienced and often medically-trained therapists), serious impulsive or risk-taking behaviour, and those seeking gratification from the therapeutic relationship, rather than insight and change.

Within the NHS, psychotherapy is usually offered once weekly, or twice weekly in exceptional circumstances, and usually for a time-limited period, typically of 9–12 months. Consultant psychotherapists offer both an assessment and supervision service to maximize the number of patients who can be appropriately placed and treated. Either individual or group psychotherapy may be offered.

Psychoanalysis

Full psychoanalysis involves five times weekly analytic psychotherapy. The patient usually reclines on a couch, with the analyst out of view, and is invited to free associate. This intensive psychotherapeutic treatment enables a full exploration of the unconscious and cognitive and behavioural restructuring. It is a feasible and appropriate treatment option for only a small number of patients, but the experience is the core training of most medically qualified psychotherapists.

Therapists may have been trained in a number of different theoretical models, a full description of which is beyond the scope of this handbook. In brief, Sigmund Freud developed the technique of free association and the concepts of transference, the Oedipal complex and ego splitting. Carl Jung developed the field of analytical psychology with the concepts of the personal and collective unconscious, archetypes and viewed treatment as a process of individuation. Melanie Klein developed the field of child analysis and the theories of primitive defence mechanisms, the paranoid–schizoid and depressive positions, and the concept of identification with idealized internal objects. Anna Freud also developed child analysis and developmental theories and elaborated on defence mechanisms. John Bowlby developed attachment theory and Winnicott the concept of object relations and the use of transitional objects. Fritz Perls developed gestalt therapy with the use of active therapeutic techniques and Carl Rogers developed client-centred therapy. For more details on these and other theoretical models the reader is advised to consult a basic psychotherapy textbook.

An assessment of a potential client may reveal a preference or aptitude for a therapist trained in a particular model.

Behavioural therapy

Behavioural treatments are practical, problem-oriented and empirically based. Treatment aims to change dysfunctional behaviours. The therapist explores with the patient the antecedents of the behaviours, full details of the behaviours themselves, and the consequences thereof, and alternative behaviours are advised to break a maladaptive pattern. Behaviours are arranged in a graded hierarchy, with an agenda set to treat problem areas in a stepwise fashion, so that gains can be seen by patients and carers and self-esteem and motivation remain high. Behavioural treatments are used to treat a number of the neuroses, in sexual dysfunction, and to bring about behavioural change in childhood disorders such as conduct disorder and hyperactivity, and in children and adults with learning difficulties and challenging behaviours. Behavioural therapy is also used as an adjunct to other treatments in chronic psychoses and affective disorders. It is most often combined with cognitive therapy.

Behavioural treatments might range from advising a stepwise increase in activity in a chronically depressed person, to techniques for remembering to take medication in dementia, which could be offered by a GP or community nurse, to complex interventions delivered by trained behavioural therapists, who could have a background in psychology, nursing or occupational therapy.

Some specific techniques are used in different disorders, such as systematic desensitization and exposure in phobias, operant conditioning or the use of rewards for desired behaviour (e.g. a star chart) in childhood disorders such as enuresis, and response prevention in obsessions. Some behaviourally-based treatment packages can be useful in a broad range of psychiatric illnesses such as relaxation techniques and social skills training. Behavioural techniques can be learned in a one-to-one therapeutic relationship, in a group, or within the dynamic of a couple or family, depending on the presenting problem.

Cognitive therapy

This is another form of problem-oriented psychological treatment. It is often used in conjunction with behavioural techniques (cognitive behavioural therapy) or with insight-oriented work (cognitive analytical therapy). It can be an alternative to pharmacological treatment (e.g. in depression) or be used as an adjunct to other treatments. In a contracted series of sessions, patients are taught a set of problem-solving techniques that enable them to gain control over their symptoms. The principles behind cognitive therapy are that an individual's behavioural and emotional responses will be shaped by their interpretation and evaluation of information from the environment; that the processing of this information is disordered in psychological disturbance and manifests as irrational beliefs; and that patients can learn to identify and change this bias in information processing which will result in symptomatic improvement.

Cognitive therapy was developed as a theoretical and practical model by Aaron Beck and colleagues in Philadelphia. There are specific cognitive models for depression, anxiety and other disorders. In depression, the cognitive triad is said to be a negative view of the self, the world, and the future and the depressed person experiences frequent negative automatic thoughts. There is often a core belief that the patient is worthless, that living is pointless. Such negative thoughts deepen depression, and lead to behavioural manifestations of low activity, social withdrawal and poor coping abilities. In anxiety there is an overestimation of threat and an underestimation of coping and support factors. The patient views him or herself as vulnerable, the world as dangerous and the future as unpredictable. In panic disorder there is a catastrophic misinterpretation of bodily sensations. There are often underlying assumptions that predispose patients to emotional disturbance, which may have arisen early in life and which act as rules for living (e.g. 'if I am not a high achiever no-one will like me'). Critical events later in life can activate these assumptions and lead to cognitive disturbances. Cognitive therapy aims to break into the vicious circles of maladaptive thinking and subsequent pathological behaviours.

The cognitive therapist and patient need to negotiate a collaborative working alliance. An assessment will be made of the presenting problems and areas of life that have been affected. These will be clarified in detail and the patient's motivations for change and reinforcements for stasis will be examined. The model of working is explained, which will include an explanation of the need for the patient to learn and work at new strategies for coping with and ultimately resolving symptoms. Some patients are unable to work with the model, if they believe that the therapist should cure them, rather than their having to learn self-help mechanisms. A clear agenda and targets will be set, homework may be given and a series of sessions will be contracted. Family and carers may become involved as therapeutic allies, particularly if behavioural work is undertaken simultaneously. The therapist is quite directive, and offers encouragement.

Specific techniques will be taught that revolve around becoming more conscious of automatic and distorted cognitions and then strategies for changing them. These include distraction techniques, thought stopping, and challenging irrational beliefs.

Cognitive, or cognitive behavioural, therapy is of proven value in depression, generalized anxiety, specific phobias, obsessional ruminations, panic disorder and in chronic pain. It is being used more widely and successes have been reported in chronic fatigue syndrome and eating disorders. It can be used as an adjunct to pharmaceuticals with an additive effect.

Like brief focused therapy, cognitive behavioural therapy appeals to purchasers of mental health care because it is time-limited and relatively inexpensive. Some GPs are purchasing specific sessions of therapy time. Therapists come from a variety of backgrounds, principally psychology.

Context of psychological treatment

It will be important to decide whether a patient receives psychological treatment as an individual, within a group, with a marital or other partner, or within the context of their family. Factors that will influence this decision are the patient's presenting problem, their preference, and the level of available resources. Individual therapy is not necessarily more expensive, especially in problem-focused treatments such as cognitive behavioural therapy, given the intensive level of therapeutic input.

Group therapy

This was first used by physicians at the turn of the century for support and teaching. Group psychotherapy was first described by Moreno around 1920, who developed the practice of psychodrama for the re-enactment of early experiences using the group as cast and audience. Group therapeutic factors have been described by Foulkes, Bion and Yalom. In essence, a group becomes a microcosm in which the group member can be confronted with the effects of his or her behaviour on others, where he or she receives support and challenge, and where the group provides a safe context in which to experiment with change. It is also possible to learn from the experiences and mistakes of others, is often a cathartic forum and social skills can be gained. Groups can be psychodynamic in orientation, self-help groups, geared towards behavioural changes (e.g. social skills training) and extend to the level of therapeutic communities.

A patient would be considered a good candidate for group therapy if they volunteer for a group rather than being coerced under pressure, if they have good verbal and conceptual skills, and if they do not view a group as inferior to individual therapy. They should have a concern with relationships or problems that can be focused in this way, they should be able to attend at a regular time (often for a longer time period than for individual work) and not be openly contemptuous. The group will need to set its own boundaries regarding confidentiality and other rules such as acceptable lateness, missed sessions, sexual tensions, etc. The facilitator's role is to manage the boundaries and anxieties, to interpret, to encourage interactions, to discourage factors impeding the group's progress and to make use of what the group brings.

Couple therapy

This is obviously of particular relevance when the presenting problem lies within the couple dynamic, whether the problem be emotional or sexual. However, couple therapy can also be useful if one partner has a particular psychiatric illness in that the 'well' partner can be co-opted as an adjunctive therapist; and also where a therapist feels that some work may need to be done as a couple to strengthen the relationship before one partner moves on to deeper individual therapy, which could involve remembering early traumas (e.g. sexual dysfunction in a marriage which a wife believes is due to her prior history of childhood sexual abuse). Couple therapy will enable the exploration of differing expectations, communication patterns and different goals. Aims should be specific, attainable and there should be a willingness to accept greater flexibility, changes in roles and responsibilities and to look for practical coping skills and solutions.

Family therapy

This is the accepted mode of service delivery in child and adolescent psychiatry. In some countries, such as Australia, most adult psychiatric illnesses are treated in a family context, at least at the level of psychoeducation and support being given so that a patient can almost always be treated in the community. In family therapy the family, rather than one individual member, is viewed as the disturbed unit. Often a team of therapists work together, with a male and female therapist in the room with the family and others behind a screen or on video–audio link. Firstly, a family is encouraged to come together to engage, and the views of different family members are sought on current problems. Agreement needs to be reached on aims and expectations of therapy and on realistic goals. The family will be encouraged to improve communication, to find new ways of resolving conflicts and will focus on interactions. Specific interventions will be used, which may be behavioural, educational or interpretive. Interventions may focus on the power balance within a family, control mechanisms and distortions, and aim at changing dysfunctional patterns.

The main theoretical models of family therapy are structural family therapy (Minuchin), systemic or Milan family therapy and strategic therapy (Haley). In all of these the role of the therapist will include encouraging family members to talk to one another rather than to the therapist, taking nothing for granted but exploring and elaboration and circular questioning. The structural family therapist will encourage enactment, reframing and changing the balance of power. A systemic therapist will look at inflexibilities, family rules and beliefs, and recurring dysfunctional patterns. A strategic therapist might view the presenting problem as a metaphor for an inflexible pattern of interaction and communication.

Although conjoint working has been described (seeing the whole family together) there are times when a collateral way of working (different therapists seeing different family members) is more appropriate. This might be particularly useful in some stages of abuse work.

Psychotherapy across cultures

There has been great concern recently that ethnic minorities have difficulty in gaining access to psychotherapy services and that such services are not culturally sensitive. Transference phenomena are likely to be problematic whenever the cultural backgrounds of therapist and patient are very dissimilar. Nafsiyat, an intercultural psychotherapy centre, has practised intercultural therapy for many years with success. The centre deliberately set itself against ethnic matching except where issues of language made it impossible. Many black organizations still suspect, and voice, that black experience cannot be understood unless the therapist has first-hand experience of being black. For example, a black patient's experience of racism may not be recognized by a non-black therapist to have had such a dramatic impact.

Further, western therapists and psychiatrists are often confused as to which is the better approach. Finite resources exclude the possibility of routinely matching client and therapist by ethnicity, yet there may be instances in which racial matching is necessary. Should the client's own preference be taken into account? Certainly there are cases where a person would wish for therapy in English despite it being their second language; similarly a refusal to see a therapist from the same ethnic group and culture has often been cited by patients in disclosure of acts or events which are, according to one's culture, taboo.

All societies have some form of schema to

make distinctions between desired and undesired states of being. They all have recognized and culturally sanctioned ways of returning an individual to a state of health. It is therefore the patient's desired modality of treatment that needs to be identified, and explanation made as to whether this can be offered or not or indeed why culturally sanctioned treatments have failed. Furthermore, assumptions cannot be made that the patient has understood the purpose of therapy and at the outset a careful explanation needs to be given about the structure of the therapy on offer and why it *might* be of help to them.

One would expect the language of therapy not to impact on the theoretical model used; one must bear in mind, however, that psychotherapy packaged as it is in the West is ethnocentric regardless of the ethnic origin of the therapist. That is not the same as saying that a black person is unable to use it, just that they have not previously had the opportunity. The requirement is therefore to take as much time as is necessary at the assessment stage to ensure that the therapist has fully understood the patient and his/her wishes and that the patient understands what is available and what demands that may entail and indeed how long they would attend for.

SOCIAL TREATMENTS

Social treatments are often listed as an afterthought in a psychiatric management plan. However, rather than being a final topping, they can be the most therapeutic interventions made, enabling a patient to minimize stresses and maximize positive benefits within their social environment. Social treatments need to be individually tailored, based on need, and should not be geared solely at the patient. Often, interventions aimed at carers, such as easing an application for attendance allowance or putting the carer in touch with a support group, prove to be the deciding factors in enabling a patient to function well within the community.

Underlying concepts

Understanding the role of the patient's social context within their illness

The social history section of a standard psychiatric clerking often consists of a mere two lines. However, a systematic analysis of the patient's place in society can yield information pertinent to aetiology, diagnosis and management. The psychiatrist or mental health team should obtain a social history, which gives clues to predisposing, precipitating and perpetuating factors in the patient's illness (e.g. predisposing: immigrant family seeking asylum; precipitating: stress over Home Office hearing; perpetuating: temporary crowded housing, financial worries, poor English) and only then can a social treatment plan be suggested.

Transcultural issues

A patient's illness, and a relevant management plan, should take account of transcultural factors. Beliefs about mental health, symptom patterns and presentation to services are all modified by the patient's cultural background, as are appropriate interventions. In particular, a mental health team will need to have a supply of leaflets printed in languages reflecting the ethnic mix of the local population, access to non-family member translators is important, and the team will need to be aware of specific local facilities for those of different cultural backgrounds. Sex and ethnicity of the allocated keyworker may be important in engaging a patient.

Multidisciplinary working

Psychiatrists rarely have a thorough working knowledge of local libraries, reductions in leisure centre entrance fees for the unemployed and evening classes. Expertise in social treatments is likely to lie with those less conditioned in the medical model, i.e. the occupational therapists and social workers within the team. In working with the long-term mentally ill, social treatments often need to be presented in a stepwise fashion, and a keyworker who is committed to continuity of care and who can act as a coordinator for a long-term plan involving ongoing assessment and input from different members of the team is essential. Keyworkers need to develop particular skills in negotiating inter-agency cooperation if a patient is to benefit fully from social interventions.

Normalization

Social treatments should aim to restore a patient to as normal a role as feasible within society, and enable them to see themselves as people who are more than their illness. To this end, social treatments aim at increasing self-esteem and obtaining a sense of mastery. Obviously, interventions that help a patient to gain skills, rather than providing others to perform tasks for them, are more beneficial. Additionally, making use of local community facilities, even if support is required for the patient to do so, is preferable to providing services which are only open to the mentally ill.

Taking account of the patient's beliefs about their social context

Patients usually have strong opinions about which social factors cause them most stress and bring on relapses, and those which keep them healthy. Social treatments cannot be prescribed – they need to be negotiated with a patient. If a patient does not see him or herself as isolated he or she will not want to attend day centres. Such treatments need to make the most of a patient's motivating factors.

Treatment within society

Social treatments cannot be delivered solely at a team base. Work may need to be done within the patient's home with their family or support network. The patient may need support from a team worker to attend a class, or visit housing options. A team also needs to hold a database of local facilities – sectorization aids the process of accumulating such knowledge.

Specific social needs

Inadequate housing

This is often a cause of major stress, particularly in deprived inner city areas. Housing may be inadequate because it is temporary (provoking anxiety), in poor repair (leading to high heating bills, unsanitary conditions, etc.), or inappropriate (within a family with high expressed emotion, unsupported, pets not allowed, unsuitable for disabled, area of high racial tension, etc.). Improving a patient's housing may simply involve a call to get a boiler fixed; informing a council or housing association tenant that they have a named housing support worker; or tracking down a maintenance department or landlord. Helping a patient with rehousing will involve an assessment of need, particularly for the level of support required (24-hour staffed, day-only cover, warden available, group home, independent living). Patients with psychiatric impairment are entitled to priority in housing allocation. Some areas have housing options available under health authority or specific mental health charity control.

Financial problems

Under community care guidelines, individuals are entitled to a needs assessment, which will involve financial review. Patients may be entitled to rebates or additional benefits (e.g. disability living allowance, grants to assist those leaving hospital). Input may be required from a debt counsellor, or training in budgeting may be needed (e.g. regular purchase of TV licence and utilities stamps, use of direct debits, etc.). For those with long-term mental illness or impairment, guardianship may need to be considered as an option to ensure adequate financial management.

Education

The proportion of school leavers without basic literacy/numeracy skills is increasing in the UK.

Those from a non-English-speaking background will also be handicapped by inability to read leaflets, fill in forms, etc. Training in such basic skills, or learning English, can be the most important intervention a team makes. For those who have missed out on education through ill health or low motivation during school years, flexible learning options, from part-time vocational courses to modular degrees, are now an option. Attendance of a class is also a valuable social opportunity.

Isolation

Isolation cannot be treated without an understanding of its cause. Social anxiety will need to be treated before a patient will be able to mix with others. Withdrawal due to depression is unlikely to improve without treatment of the depression. Those with poor English will need to be made aware of appropriate foreign language facilities. Isolation may need to be treated in a stepwise fashion, first by encouraging attendance at a team base or support group for those with similar illnesses, then by supported attendance at community facilities, then by offering options for independent socialization.

Employment

Employment offers not only financial security but also a time structure, an opportunity for social interaction, and a sense of self-esteem and identity through having a useful role. In times of high unemployment, every assistance should be given to enable a patient to remain in work. If a job has been stressful to the extent of being implicated in the aetiology of the patient's illness, stress management or relaxation techniques may be helpful in enabling the patient to cope more adequately. For a patient with a long-term relapsing illness, careful attention may need to be paid to relapse signs, so that suitable action can be taken before the patient's health deteriorates to a level which affects their work performance. Some employers are sympathetic to employees with mental illness, and may be able to support a patient if their occupational health department has a knowledge of the patient's health and illness-management plan. It may be possible to find alternative employment in a less stressful job within the same company. For those who cannot remain in their current employment, or for the unemployed, government-sponsored job clubs may be helpful in advising a patient on suitable work opportunities. Voluntary work can be a useful interim measure, or an important step on the road to job readiness. For the more disabled, employment opportunities may be forthcoming through agencies such as the disablement resettlement officer, employment rehabilitation centres, skills training centres, or through initiatives set up by local mental health charities. Local branches of MIND often run cafés and shops staffed by those recovering from mental illness. In some areas, collectives are established by community mental health teams to run print shops, catering facilities and cleaning firms, which often network with local hospitals to gain contracts. If a member of the collective becomes unwell, another member will undertake to fulfil their duties. These collectives can be an important stepping stone for those aiming to return to full-time work.

Leisure

Again, the principle of accessing local community services is all-important. Many local authorities have leisure centres, gyms, swimming pools, and activity centres that offer reduced rates to those claiming benefits. Non-vocational classes at local education centres can enable a patient to learn a new hobby or retrieve an old skill, and to meet other people simultaneously. A keyworker can also explore with the patient their desire for green spaces, via parks or day trips to the country, whether they would like to join a specific interest club, whether they would like penfriends, etc.

Transport

Those on low incomes, the mentally ill included, may be hampered in their pursuit of a full and active life by lack of money for travelling. Some local authorities are willing to give disabled-person travel passes to those suffering from mental illness. British Rail and major bus companies often have special discount schemes or offers that can lessen the expense of travelling. For those who have become very isolated, it may be necessary for a team member to pick up patients from home in order to begin a process of rehabilitation in team base activities. Also, such activities should be planned for times when cheap travel is possible (out of commuter hours) and when nervous patients will not be put off by travelling after dark.

Other sources of support

Self-help/support groups

Support groups are an important source of help for both patients and carers. They may be set up by a mental health team, or may exist locally. If set up by professionals, they are an important opportunity for psychoeducation and for building a therapeutic alliance. Through a support group, patients can learn more about how others manage illness symptoms, and feel less isolated. Carers can network to maximize their knowledge of available resources, to socialize, and to find more coping strategies. Local MIND offices will have information about support groups, and the addresses for such organizations as the Manic Depressive Fellowship, the National Schizophrenia Association, and others, are listed at the end of this handbook.

Voluntary agencies

As well as nationally known charities, many areas will have a network of voluntary agencies, and non-government organizations paid by social services, who can offer support and rehabilitation. Examples might be schemes such as Crossroads, which offers practical help to carers, respite schemes, good neighbour schemes and organizations which provide holidays for those with long-term mental illness. Local libraries should have a listing of all such agencies.

Conclusion

Social interventions should form part of any management plan in psychiatry. It is important to remember that both a patient and their family or network of friends may need support. It is also important to achieve the right balance between positive encouragement and over-enthusiastic recommendations that might overload a patient.

REFERENCES

1   Rogers, H.J. & Spector, R.G. (1984) *Aids to Clinical Pharmacology*. London: Churchill Livingstone.

2   Ashton, H. & Harrison, R. (1994) Relevance of pharmacokinetics to prescribing in psychiatry. *British Journal of Hospital Medicine* **51**, 573–580.

3   Taylor, D. *et al.* (1994) The Bethlem & Maudsley Trust prescribing guidelines. Drugs and therapeutics committee, Bethlem & Maudsley Trust.

4   Pether, R. (1993) Guidelines for the prevention and treatment of benzodiazepine dependence. *Psychiatric Bulletin* **17**, 556–557.

5   Bridges, P.K., Bartlett, J.R., Hale, A.S., Poynton, A.M., Malizia, A.L & Hodkiss, A.D. (1994) Psychosurgery: stereotactic subcaudate tractotomy. *British Journal of Psychiatry* **165**, 599–611.

Section X
Useful Information

ADDRESSES

Voluntary organizations

Action on Phobias   8 The Avenue, Eastbourne, East Sussex BN21 3YA. 01321 53227

Afro-Caribbean Mental Health Association   35–37 Electric Avenue, London SW9 8JP. 0171 737 3603

Agoraphobia Information Service 4 Manor Brook Road, London SE3 9AW. 0171 318 5026

Al-Anon   61 Great Dover Street, London SE1 4YF. 0171 403 0888. Support for relatives and families of problem drinkers (24-hour helpline)

Alcoholics Anonymous   PO Box 1, Stonebow House, Stonebow, York YO1 2NJ. 0171 352 3001

Alzheimer's Disease Society   Gordon House, 10 Greencoat Place, London SW1P 1PH. 0171 306 0606

Asian Family Counselling Service   Rooms 4/5, 40 Equity Chambers, Piccadilly, Bradford. 74 The Avenue, Ealing, London W13 8LB

Association of Carers   58 New Road, Chatham, Kent ME4 4QR

Association for Post-natal Illness 7 Gowan Avenue, London SW6 6RH. 0171 731 4867

BACUP (British Association of Cancer United Parents)   121–123 Charterhouse Street, London EC1M 6AA. 0171 608 1661

Carers National Association   29 Chilworth Mews, London W2 3RG. 0171 724 7776

Cot Death Society   7 Friars Walk, Thornby, Merseyside L37 4EU. 01704 870005

CRUSE – Bereavement Care   Cruse House, 126 Sheen Road, Richmond, Surrey TW9 1UR. 0181 940 4818

Depression Alliance   PO Box 1022, London SE1 7QB. 0171 721 7672

Eating Disorders Association   Sackville Place, 44 Magdalen Street, Norwich NR3 1JE. 01603 621414

Families Anonymous   0171 281 8889

Foundation for the Study of Infant Deaths   35 Belgrave Square, London SW1X 8QB. 0171 235 1721

Guidepost Trust   Two Rivers, Station Lane, Witney, Oxon OX8 6BH. 01993 772886 (provides supported housing)

Homestart   2 Salisbury Road, Leicester LE1 7QR. 01533 554988

Making Space   46 Allen Street, Warrington WA2 7JB. 01925 571680. Self-help and carers support in the north of England

Manic Depression Fellowship   13 Rosslyn Road, Twickenham TW1 2AR. 0181 892 2811

Mental After-Care Association   25 Bedford Square, London WC1B 3HW. 0171 436 6194

MIND   22 Harley Street, London W1N 2ED. 0171 637 0741. Produce authoritative educational materials

Nafsiyat Intercultural Therapy Centre 278 Seven Sisters Road, Finsbury Park, London N4 2HY. 0171 263 4130

Narcotics Anonymous   PO Box 1980, London N19 3LS. 0171 498 9005

National Association of Young Peoples' Counselling and Advice Services
11 Newarke Street, Leicester LE1 5SS. 01553 558763

National Black Mental Health Association   Macro House, 182 Soho Hill, Handsworth, Birmingham B19 1AF

National Council of Voluntary Organisations (NCVO)   Regent's Wharf, 8 All Saints Street, London N7 9RL. 0171 713 6161 (can provide local information)

National Schizophrenia Fellowship
28 Castle Street, Kingston upon Thames, Surrey KT1 1SS. 0181 547 3937

NEWPIN   St Margaret House, 21 Old Fort Road, London E2 9PL. 0181 980 3639

Phobic Action   Claybury Grounds, Manor Road, Woodford Green, Essex IG8 8PR. 0181 559 2551

Phobic Society   4 Cheltenham Road, Chorlton-cum-Hardy, Manchester M21 1QN. 0161 881 1937

Refugee Support Centre   King George House, Stockwell Road, London SW9 9ES. 0171 733 1482

RELATE   Herbert Grey College, Little Church St, Rugby CV21 3AP. 01788 573241

Re-Solv, Society for the Prevention of Solvent and Volatile Substance Abuse
30a High Street, Stone, Staffs ST15 8AW. 01785 817885

Richmond Fellowship for Community Mental Health   8 Addison Road, Kensington, London W14 8DL. 0171 603 6373

Samaritans   17 Uxbridge Road, Slough SL1 1SN. 01753 532713

SANE (Schizophrenia a National Emergency) 2nd Floor, 199–205 Old Marylebone Road, London NW7 5QD. 0171 724 6520

SANELINE (telephone helpline) 0171 724 8000

SCODA (Standing Committee on Drug Abuse) 1 Hatton Place, London EC1N 8ND. 0171 430 2341

Stillbirth and Perinatal Deaths Association Argyle House, 29–31 Euston Road, London NW1 2SD. 0171 833 2851

Survivors Speak Out 33 Lichfield Road, Cricklewood, London NW2

Terence Higgens Trust BM AIDS, London WC1N 3XX. 0171 242 1010

Translation services: most hospitals have registers of translators. If not, ask around staff, ask personnel, try social services, local universities

Turning Point 101 Backchurch Lane, London E1 1LU. 0171 702 2300

United Kingdom Advocacy Network The Paddocks, Haggonsfields, Rhodesia, Worksop, Notts S80 3HW

VOICES 28 Castel Street, Kingston Upon Thames, Surrey KT1 1SS. 0181 547 3939 (groups for people who have experienced schizophrenia)

Other useful addresses

British Association for Counselling 1 Regent Place, Rugby CV21 2PJ. 01788 578328. Will provide list of local counselling services; SAE required

Committee on the Safety of Medicines
Market Towers, 1 Nine Elms Lane, London
SW8 5NQ. 0171 720 2188

Home Office (Drugs Branch)   50 Queen
Annes Gate, London SW1H 9AT.
0171 273 2213

Lifeskills   3 Brighton Road, London N2 8JU.
0181 2346 9646. Offer a variety of tapes and
leaflets on mental health problems

Medical Defence Union   0171 486 6181.

Medical Protection Society
0171 637 0541

Mental Health Act Commission
01602 505040

Mental Health Foundation   8 Hallam
Street, London W1N 6DH. 0171 580 0145.
Produces a number of leaflets for the general
public on seeing a psychiatrist, the anxious
child, schizophrenia and the family, mental
handicap and the family

Royal College of Psychiatrists
17 Belgrave Square, London SW1X 8PG.
Produces a series of leaflets on depression,
anorexia, bulimia, anxiety, phobias and
bereavement

SANE Publications   199–205 Marylebone
Road, London NW1 5QP. Offer very
informative booklets for patients and carers
covering schizophrenia, depression, manic-
depression, anxiety, phobias, obsessions,
medical methods of treatment, psychological
methods of treatment, alcohol and drugs

Phenomenology

In descriptive psychopathology, items are ordered as they would be encountered in writing down the mental state examination. Within each heading, items are listed alphabetically.

Appearance and behaviour

General description of patient

What does the person look like, how are they dressed?

Abnormal postures

The general demeanour of the person is important: are they slumped in the chair sad and miserable, are they cowering fearfully in the corner, or beaming expansively at the interviewer?

Perseveration of posture is seen in schizophrenia, catalepsy and midbrain lesions.

Waxy flexibility. Seen primarily in schizophrenia, when the person stops moving they maintain a fixed posture. It is also possible to place the person in a posture which they will maintain. Unlike catatonia the muscles are not contracted.

Catatonia

Occurs in *catatonic schizophrenia* and is characterized by increased muscle tone. The person may exhibit no response to pain and may be incontinent.

Stupor

Akinetic mutism is caused by space-occupying lesions of the third ventricle, thalamus and midbrain. The patient will appear alert with eyes open, exhibit a slight response to pain and has impaired registration and recall.

Depressive stupor. There is no catalepsy or incontinence and muscle tone is normal. Stupor may also be psychogenic.

Movements

Goal-directed movements

Mannerisms are abnormal, repetitive, goal-directed movements, such as a patient's arm describing a large arc every time a fork is used to pick up a mouthful of food.

Obstruction occurs when the person requires several attempts to complete an action. Sometimes they manage it, sometimes they don't. This is seen in catatonia and schizophrenia.

Non-goal-directed movements

Athetoid movements are slow, writhing, rotatory movements particularly of the hands. The person may also assume unusual postures.

Catatonic excitement. The person shows senseless, apparently purposeless destructive behaviour whilst moving in a stilted fashion with deadpan features.

Choreiform movements are spontaneous, abrupt, random and jerky in nature and may resemble fragments of goal-directed actions. For example, someone with Huntington's chorea may be able to turn a jerky arm movement into scratching their head or it may appear as if this was the intention. These movements can involve the trunk, limbs and face. There is often also snorting- and sniffing-like actions. In Sydenham's chorea the movements are less jerky, tone is decreased and reflexes prolonged.

Gilles de la Tourette's syndrome. This begins during childhood and involves tics of movement and verbal expression. There may be limb or facial tics such as grimacing or jumping, the sufferer will make repetitive grunting or barking noises and may exhibit *coprolalia* by shouting obscenities.

Oculogyric crises can appear as an abnormal facial tic or mannerism.

Parkinsonism which may be secondary to medication.

Spasmodic torticollis involves involuntary contraction of the sternomastoids.

Stereotypies are seen in normal people, schizophrenia, mental handicap and autism. The subject will repeatedly carry out the same movement such as foot tapping or more complex actions.

Tardive dyskinesia. Secondary to antipsychotic medication. Look for orofacial dyskinesia with lip smacking and tongue movements, and limb movements. Consider also akathisia as a cause of restlessness.

Tics may appear like expressive or defensive, usually facial, movements. They are seen in dystonia, after encephalitis, Huntington's chorea and Gilles de la Tourette's syndrome.

Tremor characteristically involves the hands but may involve other parts of the body also. A resting tremor may be a normal 'essential' tremor, due to anxiety, medication (lithium), alcohol. It may be a pill-rolling tremor of parkinsonism or the characteristic lip smacking and tremor of tardive dyskinesia. Intention tremor may point to cerebellar disease.

Provoked movements

Automatic obedience is a rare feature of schizophrenia, catatonia and dementia. The subject will literally obey any command automatically.

Echopraxia. The patient copies the interviewer's or other's movements. It is seen in schizophrenia, dementia, learning difficulty, epilepsy, anxiety in small children, transcortical aphasia and delirium.

Forced grasping is a symptom of frontal lobe disease. When shaking hands, the subject repeatedly takes and holds on to the proffered hand.

Mitgehen. Seen in schizophrenia and organic brain conditions, when the subject is pushed they move freely.

Mitmachen. If the person is placed in a position they stay there.

Negativism, also called *gegenhalten*. This is seen in schizophrenia and organic brain disorders. It appears like passive resistance to movement and is not necessarily defensive or aggressive.

Mood

The themes are the constancy, appropriateness and reactivity of mood.

Depression

Look for low mood, retardation, misery, inner emptiness, hopelessness, no energy, early morning waking, weight loss, diurnal mood variation, hope for the future, ideas of self-harm.

Mania

The mood may be expansive, irritable, infectiously cheerful, decreased sleep, increased energy, increased libido.

Schizophrenia

There is great variability in mood in schizophrenia.

Flat/blunted. There is a loss of the normal range of emotions, the person seems numbed and not to react much to anything. Seen most frequently in chronic schizophrenia or when heavily medicated.

Incongruent. The mood or affect is at odds with what is being discussed or what is being described. In hebephrenic schizophrenia the affect is characteristically *fatuous*.

Perplexity, anxious puzzled bewilderment, may characterize typically the prodromal or acute stages. Alternatively the person may be very suspicious, hostile or frightened.

Other

Alexithymia (literally, no words to feel). Some people find it almost impossible to describe their emotions in words.

Denial is a defence mechanism and is often a normal reponse. It is not the same as incongruent affect or the coldness of psychopathy.

Emotional indifference. This is an extreme form of denial also known as *belle indifference*. Typically the person in hospital with a conversion disorder that leaves them paralysed will not seem at all bothered as staff try to establish the cause.

Emotional incontinence involves extreme lability of mood from moment to moment. It can be associated with organic conditions such as frontal lobe syndromes or pseudobulbar palsy.

Lability. Occurs in mania, personality disorder, and organic conditions.

Speech and thought

Specific psychiatric disorders have typical disorders of the form and content of speech associated with them. These constellations of signs and symptoms are not pathognomonic but are indicative.

Korsakoff

Confabulation. Asked what they had for breakfast that morning or for details of past psychiatric history, patients will tell a more or less plausible story that is completely invented.

Mania

Pressure of speech, rhyming, punning, flight of ideas.

Flight of ideas is considered here for convenience. There is a loss of coherent goal-directed thinking with only obscure connections between ideas. It is possible to trace the train of ideas unlike loosening of associations.

Pressure of speech. It is not possible to interrupt the stream of talk. Attempts to do so are ignored, talked over, met with irritability.

Rhyming. The patient will inventively rhyme their speech; may also use assonance and alliteration (clang associations).

Organic

Some symptoms are strongly indicative of an organic brain disorder.

Dysarthria. A disturbance of the articulation of speech due to muscle dysfunction.

Dysphasia. A disturbance of either the comprehension (receptive) or expression of speech most commonly due to a cerebrovascular disorder.

Echolalia. Heard speech is repeated, usually only a word or phrase.

Palilalia is indicative of organic brain disorder. A perseverated word is repeated faster and often.

Perseveration. A single word is repeated over and over again. It is not a stereotypy because the word was relevant to its context but persisted.

Logoclonia. A single syllable is repeated over and over, usually the last syllable of the last word. Seen in Parkinson's disease.

Verbigeration is a form of verbal stereotypy. Sentences, phrases or jargon are repeated for hours on end.

Schizophrenia

In acute schizophrenia there are a number of different approaches to discussing formal thought disorder. Bleuler described schizophrenia as a disorder of associations of which loosening of associations is a manifestation. Schneider characterized schizophrenic thought disorder differently. He described five features (derailment, omission, substitution, fusion and drivelling) which come together to make three patterns: transitory, desultory and drivelling thinking. In addition there are other terms used to describe other aspects of schizophrenic thought disorder.

Bleuler

Loosening of associations. Bleuler used this term to describe condensation, displacement and the concrete use of symbols in schizophrenia.

Condensation is the incomprehensible combination of two or more ideas. It is difficult to distinguish from derailment and 'knight's move' thinking.

Schneider

Derailment. Disrupted continuity and insertion of inappropriate material.

Drivelling. Muddling of elements within an idea.

Fusion. Merging and intertwining of ideas.

Omission of part or a whole thought.

Substitution. The main stream of thought is replaced by a secondary one.

These five elements come together as:

Transitory thinking. Grammar and syntax are both affected.

Desultory thinking. Grammar and syntax are correct but sudden ideas force their way into the stream of talk.

Drivelling thinking. Parts of ideas become muddled up and the subject tries to unpick this.

Other aspects

Concrete thinking. A loss of the capacity for abstract thought; everything is taken very literally. One patient asked another 'Where are you from?' The other considered this for a moment and then replied 'I suppose I'm from my mother's tummy' and pointed at his abdomen to illustrate the point.

Knight's move. See derailment and loosening of associations.

Neologisms. The invention of new words or the attribution of new meanings to existing words. A patient described how people 'put the shine' on him. This neologistic use of 'shine' described how people read his thoughts and controlled his actions.

Poverty of thought. Often encountered with blunted affect and concrete thinking when negative symptoms are prominent.

Thought block. The sensation of the mind going blank is normal under stress, e.g. examinations. In thought block the sensation is of the train of thought 'hitting a brick wall' or being suddenly arrested.

Word salad. Meaningless verbigeration as the name describes.

Other disorders of speech and thinking

Mutism. Occurs in children, dissociative (conversion) disorder, depression, schizophrenia and organic syndromes.

Vorberieden. Talking past the point is seen in Ganser's syndrome and acute schizophrenia.

Obsessive–compulsive phenomena

Obsessions are impulses and thoughts, whilst compulsions are their motor accompaniment. *Obsessions* appear against the subject's will, they are recognized as a product of one's own mind, and resisting them initially increases anxiety. Resistance decreases with time. They may take the form of words, thoughts or images; their content may be sexual, religious, contamination, depressive, aggressive or about illness. They occur in depression, obsessive–compulsive disorder, schizophrenia, and after encephalitis. They involve a single thought or image repeated over and over again. Rumination involves worrying around a subject.

Abnormal beliefs, perceptions and experiences

Disorders of self-awareness

Anosognosia. Denial or lack of awareness of paralysis or sensory deficit.

Depersonalization. The sensation that one is not real or not really there. It occurs in anxiety states, schizophrenia, epilepsy, depression and organic disorders.

Derealization involves the sense that one's surroundings are dull, flat and somehow not real.

Distorted body image. In anorexia the sufferers believe themselves to be overweight, typically with 'enormous thighs' when they are actually emaciated. Some debate whether or not this is a delusion.

Delusions

Strictly these are 'disorders of the content of thought' but are always considered here when presenting the mental state.

What is the form?

Primary delusions (synonyms: autochthonous delusions and delusional perception). The experience comes out of the blue in a two-stage process where a real perception or memory is suddenly invested with a delusional meaning. It may be preceded by a delusional mood. For example, a man went into a café. The person at the next table ordered macaroni cheese. The man who had been perplexed for some time suddenly realized there was a homosexual conspiracy run by freemasons in the café. Primary delusions are a first-rank symptom of schizophrenia.

Secondary delusions derive from previous experiences; their onset is usually more insidious. They may relate to auditory hallucinations.

Over time they can become systematized into an integrated set of beliefs. They are fixed, firm, unshakeable beliefs held in the face of evidence to the contrary and out of keeping with the subject's experience and context.

Is it systematized or unsystematized?

Systematized delusions are elaborated into a consistent world view by the subject. Unsystematized delusions do not 'fit' or have the same permanence. Circumscribed delusional systems may be held in such a way that the subject's lifestyle is not interfered with at all.

What is the content?

Persecutory, grandiose, delusion of reference, erotic, religious, depressive, nihilistic, bizarre.

Overvalued ideas

These are intense preoccupations in which the subject has an emotional investment. They are not unshakeable and are demonstrably false but understandable.

Passivity phenomena

These are disorders of the possession of thought and involve loss of the sense of boundaries between the self and the world.

Made actions. The subject's physical actions are under external control: the sense is of being radio-controlled or having to respond in a particular way when a certain external event occurs.

Thought broadcast. This is an example of the loss of self boundaries. The subject experiences their thoughts being available to other people. They may appear over the radio or via television aerials.

Thought insertion. An outside agency puts alien thoughts into the subject's mind.

Thought withdrawal. Thoughts are removed as if by a vacuum cleaner. This can be differentiated from thought block by asking: 'Do you ever find that your thoughts stop dead and leave your mind a complete blank?' (thought block) and 'Do you ever find that people can interfere with your thoughts or read your mind?' (passivity).

Perceptual disturbances

Sensory distortions
These are distortions of existing perceptions.

Dysmegalopsia. Distortion of spatial form occurring with retinal scarring and temporal lobe disorders.

Hyperacusis. Extreme sensitivity to sounds as in mania and hyperthyroidism.

Hypoacusis occurs in delirium.

Micropsia. Things appear smaller than they are.

Xanthopsia. Changes in colour vision, usually drug induced. May also occur in temporal lobe epilepsy and erythopsia from retinal haemorrhage.

Sensory deceptions

Eidetic imagery. Vivid visual recall of previous perception usually occurring in the mind's eye: 'photographic memory'.

Illusions are misperceptions of external events such as seeing a tree in the dark and thinking it is a person. Seeing lines on wallpaper turn into snakes in delirium tremens is also an example of this.

Pareidolia. A type of illusion in which pictures are seen in the fire or in the clouds. It implies the creation of vivid mental images without effort.

Pseudohallucinations. This term is used in two ways. Jaspers used it to describe vivid mental images, a form of eidetic imagery or variant of fantasy. The perception is located in the mind not in external space and is not consciously manipulated. Hare used the term to describe perceptions in the absence of an external perception, which nonetheless appear to be located in the real world but which the subject recognizes as not real.

Hallucinations

A perception (or sensory deception) occurring in the *absence* of an external stimulus. They are perceived as if occurring in the real world and thus have the same qualities as real perceptions. They occur in schizophrenia, mood disorders, dissociative states, delirium, dementia, other brain disorders and in normal people. They may be formed or unformed and in any sensory modality. Obtaining a description of a hallucination is rather like getting a patient to describe a pain or a lump: what modality is it, formed or unformed, if voices one or several, strangers or familiar voices, where are they located, what are they saying, what is its effect, etc.

Auditory. May be elementary with fragments of sounds or music or voices or fully formed. In psychotic depression they are usually in the second person and derogatory or urging the person to harm themselves. In schizophrenia they are characteristically *third person,* discussing or providing a running commentary although second person voices also occur. Voices may provide a *running commentary* on the subject. *Thought echo* is a first-rank symptom of schizophrenia. It is a type of auditory hallucination in which the subject reports hearing their thoughts echoed inside their head or outside it.

Autoscopy. The ability to step outside one's body and see oneself. It can occur in extreme anxiety but is more commonly associated with intoxication with alcohol or drugs, delirium and epilepsy. In the myth of the *doppelgänger* it is part of a near-death experience.

Extracampine hallucinations occur outside the sensory field. One is able to see and hear people in another town.

Functional hallucination. A stimulus in one modality causes a hallucination; both are experienced. A woman reported hearing God talking to her when the clock chimed. It occurs in schizophrenia.

Pain and deep sensation. Twisting and tearing sensations inside the body occur in chronic schizophrenia. *Delusional zoopathy* is the sensation that an animal is living inside one's body. It can occur in pellagra, thalamic tumours and schizophrenia.

Reflex hallucination. An event perceived in one sensory modality leads to a consequence in another. When sneezing, the patient experiences a pain in the leg.

Taste and smell. Hallucinations in these modalities are rare and occur in temporal lobe epilepsy, irritation of the olfactory bulb, schizophrenia and delirium.

Touch. Formication is the sensation of having insects crawling in or under the skin. It is also called delusional infestation and can be caused by cocaine or alcohol withdrawal. The cocaine bug consists of formication plus persecutory delusions.

Vestibular hallucinations produce the sensation of flying through the air or falling back through the bed. They occur in normal people, substance abuse and intoxication and psychosis and delirium.

Visual. May be elementary (flashes), partly organized (patterns) or fully organized. They are found in delirium, dissociative states, substance abuse and other brain disorders. Lilliputian hallucinations are pleasant visual hallucinations of little people or objects that occur in delirium. LSD produces sensory distortions such as synaesthesia where one can, for example, hear colours rather than hallucinations.

Insight

This has many components beyond attitude to treatment and diagnosis. It includes recognition of illness and awareness that mental illness is a plausible explanation for present experiences. The patient should also be asked about their views of the value of compliance and the implications of their illness and its effects on self and others.

PSYCHIATRIC RATING SCALES

Standardized instruments are commonly used in psychiatric research and practice for identifying psychiatric 'cases', improving the accuracy of assessment and diagnosis, assessing the severity of psychiatric symptoms and social disabilities, and evaluating change in response to specific interventions.

There are three main types of instrument: (i) self-report, (ii) interview based and (iii) observational assessments. The choice between these depends on the purpose for which it is intended, the condition under investigation, the setting in which the study will take place, the nature of the information to be gathered, the sample size, and the time and resources available for data collection. If an interview-based measure is to be used, a further choice must be made between an instrument suitable for use by lay interviewers and one which requires specialist clinical skills.

The psychometric properties of psychiatric instruments can be considered under the headings of reliability and validity. Since there are no 'gold standards' by which to assess the validity of psychiatric instruments, great store has been set by developing instruments that are reliable. It must be remembered that while important, reliability is really of secondary significance: it is necessary but not sufficient for establishing the validity of an instrument.

Reliability refers to the repeatability of measurement. A reliable instrument is one which produces the same results on repeated administration. There are three formal criteria by which the reliability of instruments is traditionally assessed: *inter-rater* (the level of agreement between two raters), *test–retest* (agreement

X: USEFUL INFORMATION

between scores for the same subject over time), and *split-half reliability* (a measure of the internal consistency of an instrument).

Validity is defined as the extent to which an instrument measures what it claims to measure. There are five main types of validity: *face validity* (the general appearance of the instrument), *content validity* (whether an instrument appears to be a balanced and comprehensive measure of the phenomenon of interest), *criterion validity* (a measure of agreement between an instrument and an external criterion), *construct validity* (the extent to which results obtained using an instrument are consistent with theoretical assumptions underlying its design) and *predictive validity* (the extent to which scores on an instrument are predictive of some future event).

Instruments in common use

Case finding

The aims of epidemiological investigation include estimating the frequency and distribution of disorder in populations, and searching for potential aetiological risk factors. Any such enquiry requires a definition of 'caseness', and instruments capable of accurately identifying 'cases'. It must be remembered, however, that most populations contain subjects with symptoms ranging from the transient and minor to the severe and chronic, and any definition of 'caseness' amounts to the imposition of a threshold value on a continuous distribution. The current definition of a 'case' of psychiatric disorder is that the patient's symptoms fulfil the operational criteria of DSM-IV or ICD-10.

The most widely used case-finding instrument in the UK is the *General Health Questionnaire (GHQ)*.[1] The GHQ was developed on the assumption that there are undifferentiated subjective experiences of psychiatric disorder which distinguish all such patients from those who are well. The questionnaire was originally intended for use in primary-care settings, and enquires about recent changes in functioning. The resulting score is a quantitative assessment of the likelihood that an individual would be identified as a psychiatric case by a psychiatrist. The GHQ is highly acceptable to the general population, and has been extensively validated.

An alternative is the *Self-Reporting Questionnaire (SRQ)*,[2] a 24-item questionnaire developed by the WHO for use in developing countries. The SRQ is as effective in case detection as the GHQ, and yes/no response categories make it particularly suitable in settings where literacy may be poor.

Assessment of global psychopathology

The *Present State Examination (PSE)* was first published in 1967,[3] and has now reached its tenth edition. A computer program, CATEGO, was developed in 1971 to produce standardized diagnostic groupings. The PSE is designed for use by psychiatrists after a specified period of training. Interviewers are trained to discover whether each of a comprehensive list of symptoms is present, and if so with what degree of severity. For most symptoms questions are suggested, but interviewers are free to clarify with their own supplementary questions when necessary. For the ninth edition of the PSE an index of definition (ID) was constructed based on the number, type and severity of symptoms elicited. The index specifies eight levels of definition of disorder, and the threshold for 'caseness' is set between levels 4 and 5.

PSE 10 has been incorporated into the *Schedule for Clinical Assessment in Neuropsychiatry (SCAN)*.[4] SCAN represents a comprehensive procedure for clinical examination capable of generating ICD-10, DSM-III-R and DSM-IV categories. A major addition to PSE 10 is the inclusion of sections on eating disorders, somatoform disorders and alcohol and substance abuse, which were absent from PSE 9. SCAN contains a 59-item group checklist, consisting of groups of symptoms, and a clinical information schedule for use with case records, carers and other informants. SCAN also gives the option of supplementing information on present state by rating a secondary period, which can be a previous representative episode of illness or a lifetime rating.

The *Composite International Diagnostic Interview (CIDI)* is a standardized instrument designed for use by lay interviewers in epidemiological studies in cross-cultural settings.[5] The CIDI combines items from the PSE and the *Diagnostic Interview Schedule (DIS)*,[6] an instrument used by lay interviewers in the Epidemiological Catchment Area study. Data gathered using the CIDI are sufficient to make reliable ICD-10 and DSM-III-R diagnoses. Both the DIS and CIDI ask first about lifetime prevalence of symptoms, before enquiring about timing of onset and duration to arrive at lifetime, 1-year, 6-month and 3-month prevalence rates. The main advantages of CIDI are its standardization, extensive field testing in diverse settings and languages, and exceptionally high reliability. The main drawbacks of the CIDI are the time needed for training and the duration of interview, which lasts for over 2 hours in one-third of interviews.

The *Clinical Interview Schedule (CIS)*[7] was the first standardized interview designed to assess common mental disorders in community settings, among subjects who may not see themselves as psychiatrically disturbed. In its original form, the CIS resembled a clinical interview and required the interviewer to judge whether the subject was a psychiatric case, and to decide on an appropriate diagnosis. High reliability was obtained among trained raters. The CIS has been revised (*CIS-R*) for use by lay interviewers,[8] by removing all but the standardized enquiry into non-psychotic symptoms. Elimination of the 'manifest abnormality' section means that it is largely free from observer bias and less dependent on training. While extending its applicability in non-psychiatric settings, these changes did not alter the validity of the CIS. A computerized version of this instrument has been shown to possess psychometric properties similar to the original.

The *Brief Psychiatric Rating Scale (BPRS)*[9] was designed to assess treatment efficacy in psychopharmacological research, and has been used most widely among patients with psychotic disorders. The BPRS consists of 18 symptom constructs rated on a seven-point scale of severity. Reliability is high among clinically experienced raters within centres, but lack of cues for rating severity leads to variation between centres. The most serious drawbacks are the overlap between items and their lack of correspondence with current psychopathological concepts, making ratings susceptible to the halo effect.

The *Schedule for Affective Disorders and Schizophrenia (SADS)*[10] is a semi-structured interview for use by experienced clinicians and was the most widely used diagnostic instrument in psychiatric research in the USA prior to the advent of DSM-III. This interview was designed for use with psychiatric patients, and provides a comprehensive assessment of the symptoms of disorders defined by the Research Diagnostic Criteria (RDC). The full SADS interview enquires separately about the time of maximum symptom severity during the current episode, the severity of symptoms in the past week, and lifetime experience of symptoms. Other versions of the SADS include the SADS-L (lifetime version) and the SADS-C (change version) which is suitable for repeated administration with the same subject.

The *Structured Interview for DSM-III-R (SCID)*[11] is a DSM-III-R compatible version of the SADS that requires less training than the original. Unlike the SADS, the SCID incorporates diagnostic algorithms within the interview. Questions are grouped by diagnosis, and if any criterion essential to a diagnosis is not met the interviewer is instructed to skip the remaining questions about that diagnosis. Like the SADS, interviewers are encouraged to gather information from as many sources as possible. Versions of the SCID include SCID-II, which assesses personality disorders, SCID-P (patient), a self-report version for use among those identified as psychiatric patients, and SCID-NP (non-patient), for use where subjects are not necessarily seeking help for psychiatric disorders.

Assessment of the severity of specific conditions

Depression
More instruments have been developed for the assessment of depression than for any other psy-

chiatric disorder; a recent review[12] identified over 30 in the English language alone. Of these, the most commonly used are listed below.

The *Hamilton Rating Scale for Depression (HRSD)*,[13] an observer scale consisting of 17 (or, less commonly, 21) items scored on a combination of five- and three-point scales. Designed for use by experienced clinicians, training in the use of this instrument is necessary. There are no standardized questions, but a detailed glossary is provided. The instrument assesses cognitive and behavioural aspects of depression but places particular emphasis on somatic symptoms.

The *Beck Depression Inventory (BDI)*[14] is a 21-item self-report measure that assesses sadness, anhedonia, suicidal ideation, negative cognitions and somatic manifestations of depression. Like the HRSD, the BDI should only be used to assess severity once a diagnosis of depression has been made. No training in its use is necessary, and it is suitable for frequent use on the same subject.

The *Montgomery–Asberg Depression Rating Scale (MADRS)*[15] was designed to assess change in severity of depression. The MADRS consists of 10 items, none of which concerns somatic or psychomotor symptoms.

The *Hospital Anxiety and Depression Scale (HAD)*[16] was originally intended for use in general medical settings, where scores on other instruments may be contaminated by symptoms of physical illness. The HAD comprises two seven-item self-report scales. Items on the depression scale are largely restricted to the assessment of anhedonia, though anxiety items enquire about autonomic symptoms. The HAD should be used with care in applications other than that for which it was designed.

Eating disorders

The *Eating Attitudes Test (EAT)*[17] is a self-report instrument consisting of 26 items covering both cognition and behaviour. EAT score is dominated by a 'dieting' component, making it difficult to interpret except among those who are thin or pathologically preoccupied with their weight.[18] Although validated as a measure of the severity of anorexia nervosa, the EAT has also been used inappropriately for case identification in community surveys. Used in this way, the EAT has a positive predictive value of around 10%, since the prevalence of this disorder is less than 1%. The EAT is further limited by the tendency of anorexic subjects to deny their illness.

Personality disorder

The *Eysenck Personality Inventory (EPI)*[19] is the personality questionnaire most widely used in Britain. Its 48 questions measure two major orthogonal factors: extraversion/introversion (E) and neuroticism (N). The test also incorporates a lie scale. Twin studies demonstrate that both E and N are moderately heritable.

Standardized interviews based on the operational definitions of personality disorder found in ICD-10 and DSM-IV such as the *Personality Assessment Schedule (PAS)*[20] and the *Standardised Assessment of Personality (SAP)*[21] have allowed systematic research into the prevalence rate of personality disorders, their impact upon outcome for other clinical disorders, and the validity of the various subcategories of personality disorder.

Instruments used in social psychiatry

Assessment of social functioning

Social disabilities associated with psychiatric disorder can be more distressing for a patient than specific symptoms. Social impairments may be longer lasting and harder to treat, and social functioning may be a better predictor of service utilization and cost of care than either diagnosis or symptomatology.

The *Global Assessment of Functioning Scale (GAF)* was introduced as axis V of DSM-III-R, to provide a measure of 'a person's psychological, social, and occupational functioning'.[22] The GAF is a modified version of the *Global Assessment Scale (GAS)*,[23] which has been widely used in both research and clinical settings, and has established reliability. Using nine anchor points describing different levels of symptoms and functioning the rater decides on a single number between 0 and 90 to summarize a person's overall condition. Though simple, combining symptoms and functioning in a single rating may be misleading or uninformative.

A more precise measure of current functioning is obtained by examining a person's recent performance in specific social roles. The *MRC Social Role Performance Schedule (SRP)*[24] compares individual functioning with population norms, though it must be remembered that some roles may be inappropriate for certain study populations. For instance, prisoners or institutionalized patients will not have the opportunity to fulfil domestic, sexual or financial roles. The *Social Behaviour Scale (SBS)*[25] measures a range of behaviours, mainly on five-point scales, and has established psychometric properties.

Other measures relevant to psychiatry

Quality of life

Quality of life is notoriously difficult to define. The major components are the absence of symptoms, adequate social performance, and the ability to engage in satisfying activities. Two examples of quality of life measures suitable for people with mental disorders are the *Quality of Life Interview*[26] and the *Lancashire Quality of Life Schedule*.[27]

Needs assessment

People with serious mental illness frequently have a complex mix of medical and social needs. In the UK, recent government policy has placed great emphasis on the assessment of individual need, prior to the planning and delivery of care. Regular clinical assessments of patients' needs are essential for the appropriate targeting of care. Measurement of met and unmet need is a powerful outcome measure for any mental health service evaluation. The *MRC Needs for Care Assessment (NCA)* identifies potentially remediable areas in which a patient's level of functioning is at or below a minimum specified level.[24] The *Camberwell Assessment of Need (CAN)*[28] is a more recently developed instrument, which is briefer than the NCA and is suitable for use by untrained raters. This instrument covers 22 social and clinical needs. Levels of met and unmet need are recorded, along with measures of the amount of help received from informal carers and health professionals. Each item is rated independently by the subject and their keyworker.

REFERENCES

1   Goldberg, D.P. (1972) *Detecting Psychiatric Illness by Questionnaire.* Maudsley Monograph 22. Oxford: Oxford University Press.

2   Harding, T.W., de Arango, M.V., Baltazar, J. et al. (1980) Mental disorders in primary health care: a study of their frequency and diagnosis in four developing countries. *Psychological Medicine* **10**, 231–241.

3   Wing, J.K., Birley, J.L.T., Cooper, J.E. et al. (1967) Reliability of a procedure for measuring and classifying 'present psychiatric state'. *British Journal of Psychiatry* **113**, 499–515.

4   Wing, J.K., Babor,T., Brugha, T. et al. (1990) SCAN. *Archives of General Psychiatry* **47**, 589–593.

5   Robins, L.N. & Sartorius, N. (1993) Editorial. *International Journal of Methods in Psychiatric Research* **3**, 63–65.

6   Robins, L.N., Helzer, J.E., Croughan, J. et al. (1981) National Institute of Mental Health Diagnostic Interview Schedule: its history, characteristics and validity. *Archives of General Psychiatry* **38**, 381–389.

7   Goldberg, D.P., Cooper, B., Eastwood, M.R. et al. (1970) A standardised psychiatric interview for use in community settings. *British Journal of Preventive and Social Medicine* **24**, 18–23.

8   Lewis, G., Pelosi, A.J., Araya, R. et al. (1992) Measuring psychiatric disorder in the community: a standardised assessment for use by lay interviewers. *Psychological Medicine* **22**, 465–486.

9   Overall, J.E. & Gorham, D.R. (1962) The Brief Psychiatric Rating Scale (BPRS). *Psychological Reports* **10**, 799–812.

10 Endicott, J. & Spitzer, R.L. (1978) A diagnostic interview: the Schedule for Affective Disorders and Schizophrenia. *Archives of General Psychiatry* **35**, 837–844.

11 Spitzer, R.L., Williams, J.B.W., Gibbon, M. et al. (1992) The Structured Clinical Interview for DSM-III-R (SCID). I: History, rationale and description. *Archives of General Psychiatry* **49**, 624–629.

12 Snaith, P. (1993) What do depression rating scales measure? *British Journal of Psychiatry* **163**, 293–298.

13 Hamilton, M. (1960) A rating scale for depression. *Journal of Neurology, Neurosurgery and Psychiatry* **23**, 56–62.

14 Beck, A.T., Ward, C.H., Mendelson, M. et al. (1961) An inventory for measuring depression. *Archives of General Psychiatry* **4**, 561–571.

15 Montgomery, S.A. & Asberg, M. (1979) A new depression scale designed to be sensitive to change. *British Journal of Psychiatry* **134**, 382–389.

16 Zigmond, A.S. & Snaith, R.P. (1982) The Hospital Anxiety and Depression Scale. *Acta Psychiatrica Scandinavica* **67**, 361–370.

17 Garner, D.M. & Garfinkel, P.E. (1979) The Eating Attitudes Test: an index of the symptoms of anorexia nervosa. *Psychological Medicine* **9**, 273–279.

18 Wells, J.E. Cooper, P.A., Gabb, D.C. & Pears, P.K. (1985) The factor structure of the eating attitudes test with adolescent schoolgirls. *Psychological Medicine* **15**, 141–146.

19 Eysenck, H.J. and Eysenck, S.B.G. (1964) *Manual of Eysenck Personality Inventory.* London: University of London Press.

20 Tyrer, P. & Alexander, J. (1979) Classification of personality disorder. *British Journal of Psychiatry* **135**, 163–167.

21 Mann, A.H., Jenkins, R. & Cutting, J.C. (1981) The development and use of a standardised assessment of abnormal personality. *Psychological Medicine* **11**, 839–847.

22 American Psychiatric Association (1987) DSM-III-R. In UK available from The Press Syndicate, University of Cambridge, Trumpington St, Cambridge CB2 1RP.

23 Endicott, J., Spitzer, R.L., Fleiss, J.L. *et al.* (1976) The global assessment scale. *Archives of General Psychiatry* **33**, 766–771.

24 Brewin, C., Wing, J., Mangen, S. *et al.* (1987) Principles and practice of measuring needs in the long-term mentally ill: the MRC Needs of Care Assessment. *Psychological Medicine* **17**, 971–982.

25 Wykes, T. & Sturt, E. (1986) The measurement of social behaviour in psychiatric patients: an assessment of the reliability and validity of the SBS schedule. *British Journal of Psychiatry* **148**, 1–11.

26 Lehman, A. (1982) The well-being of chronic mental patients – assessing their quality of life. *Archives of General Psychiatry* **40**, 369–374.

27 Oliver, J.P.J. (1991) The Social Care Directive: development of a quality of life profile for use in community services for the mentally ill. *Social Work and Social Science Review* **3**, 5–45.

28 Thornicroft, G., Ward, P. & James, S. (1993) Care management and mental health. *British Medical Journal* **20**, 768–771.

Index

Numbers in bold refer to main reference

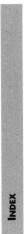

– D –

–O–

–P–

–Q–